AF886667

UNDERSTANDING

Genomic and Hereditary Cancer Risk

A HANDBOOK FOR ONCOLOGY NURSES

By
Suzanne M. Mahon, DNS, RN, AOCN®, AGN-BC, FAAN

ONS Publications Department
Publisher and Director of Publications: William A. Tony, BA, CQIA
Senior Editorial Manager: Lisa M. George, MPH, BA, CHES
Acquisitions Editor: John Zaphyr, BA, MEd
Staff Editor: Andrew Petyak, BA
Associate Staff Editor: Casey S. Kennedy, BA
Design and Production Administrator: Dany Sjoen
Editorial Assistant: Rachel Geffrey, BFA

Copyright © 2021 by the Oncology Nursing Society. All rights reserved. No part of the material protected by this copyright may be reproduced or utilized in any form, electronic or mechanical, including photocopying, recording, or by an information storage and retrieval system, without written permission from the copyright owner. For information, visit www.ons.org/publications-journals/permissions-archives, or send an email to pubpermissions@ons.org.

Library of Congress Cataloging-in-Publication Data

Names: Mahon, Suzanne M., author. | Oncology Nursing Society, issuing body.

Title: Understanding genomic and hereditary cancer risk : a handbook for oncology nurses / by Suzanne M. Mahon.
Description: Pittsburgh, Pennsylvania : Oncology Nursing Society, [2021] | Includes bibliographical references and index.
Identifiers: LCCN 2021004859 (print) | LCCN 2021004860 (ebook) | ISBN 9781635930498 (paperback) | ISBN 9781635930504 (ebook)
Subjects: MESH: Neoplasms--genetics | Genetic Predisposition to Disease | Medical History Taking | Genetic Testing | Genetic Counseling | Nurses Instruction
Classification: LCC RC268.4 (print) | LCC RC268.4 (ebook) | NLM QZ 202 | DDC 616.99/4042--dc23
LC record available at https://lccn.loc.gov/2021004859
LC ebook record available at https://lccn.loc.gov/2021004860

Publisher's Note

This book is published by the Oncology Nursing Society (ONS). ONS neither represents nor guarantees that the practices described herein will, if followed, ensure safe and effective patient care. The recommendations contained in this book reflect ONS's judgment regarding the state of general knowledge and practice in the field as of the date of publication. The recommendations may not be appropriate for use in all circumstances. Those who use this book should make their own determinations regarding specific safe and appropriate patient care practices, taking into account the personnel, equipment, and practices available at the hospital or other facility at which they are located. The author and publisher cannot be held responsible for any liability incurred as a consequence from the use or application of any of the contents of this book. Figures and tables are used as examples only. They are not meant to be all-inclusive, nor do they represent endorsement of any particular institution by ONS. Mention of specific products and opinions related to those products do not indicate or imply endorsement by ONS. Websites mentioned are provided for information only; the hosts are responsible for their own content and availability. Unless otherwise indicated, dollar amounts reflect U.S. dollars.

ONS publications are originally published in English. Publishers wishing to translate ONS publications must contact ONS about licensing arrangements. ONS publications cannot be translated without obtaining written permission from ONS. (Individual tables and figures that are reprinted or adapted require additional permission from the original source.) Because translations from English may not always be accurate or precise, ONS disclaims any responsibility for inaccuracies in words or meaning that may occur as a result of the translation. Readers relying on precise information should check the original English version.

Printed in the United States of America

ONS®
Oncology Nursing Society

Innovation • Excellence • Advocacy

DISCLOSURE

Editors and authors of books and guidelines provided by the Oncology Nursing Society are expected to disclose to the readers any significant financial interest or other relationships with the manufacturer(s) of any commercial products.

A vested interest may be considered to exist if a contributor is affiliated with or has a financial interest in commercial organizations that may have a direct or indirect interest in the subject matter. A "financial interest" may include, but is not limited to, being a shareholder in the organization; being an employee of the commercial organization; serving on an organization's speakers bureau; or receiving research funding from the organization. An "affiliation" may be holding a position on an advisory board or some other role of benefit to the commercial organization. Vested interest statements appear in the front matter for each publication.

Contributors are expected to disclose any unlabeled or investigational use of products discussed in their content. This information is acknowledged solely for the information of the readers.

The author provided the following disclosure and vested interest information:

The author had no relevant information to disclose.

LICENSING OPPORTUNITIES

The Oncology Nursing Society (ONS) produces some of the most highly respected educational resources in the field of oncology nursing, including ONS's award-winning journals, books, online courses, evidence-based resources, core competencies, videos, and information available on the ONS website at www.ons.org. ONS welcomes opportunities to license reuse of these intellectual properties to other organizations.

Licensing opportunities include the following:

- **Reprints**—Purchase high-quality reprints of ONS journal articles, book chapters, and other content directly from ONS, or obtain permission to produce your own reprints.
- **Translations**—Translate and then resell or share ONS resources internationally.
- **Integration**—Purchase a license to incorporate ONS's oncology-specific telephone triage protocols or other resources into your institution's EMR or EHR system.
- **Cobranding**—Display your company's logo on ONS resources for distribution to your organization's employees or customers.
- **Educational reuse**—Supplement your staff or student educational programs using ONS resources.
- **Customization**—Customize ONS intellectual property for inclusion in your own products or services.
- **Bulk purchases**—Buy ONS books and online courses in high quantities to receive great savings compared to regular pricing.

As you read through the pages of this book, think about whether any of these opportunities are the right fit for you as you consider reusing ONS content—and the contents of this book—for your organization.

Contact licensing@ons.org with your licensing questions or requests.

Table of Contents

Preface

Collecting a family medical history is a regular component of the nursing assessment process. Patients with cancer often report that multiple family members have been diagnosed with cancer or express concern that other family members might be at increased risk for developing cancer.

As the involvement of genetics and genomics in oncology continues to grow, so too does public awareness of hereditary risk for developing cancer. This increasing awareness directly affects oncology nursing care. Although true germline (inherited) risk for developing cancer is much less common than somatic (acquired) risk for developing cancer, approximately 10% of cancer diagnoses can be attributed to germline risk. The identification of these families enables those at increased risk to engage in increased surveillance and, in some cases, risk-reducing surgery and other preventive measures, which ultimately lead to decreasing the morbidity and mortality associated with a cancer diagnosis.

In the past two decades, genetic testing for germline risk has greatly advanced. Genetic testing in oncology practice is being utilized more frequently and is best managed by genetics professionals. Genetics professionals, however, rely on healthcare providers to identify and refer patients for evaluation. Each time nurses extract a family history, they have an opportunity to assess for possible genetic risk and, when appropriate, refer patients and families to a genetics professional for further evaluation.

This book provides background on basic genetic and genomic concepts, especially related to germline risk for developing cancer. Nurses need this information to know when and why to refer patients. Nurses also need to give patients reliable information about how and why genetic and genomic testing can not only guide treatment decisions but also guide recommendations for cancer prevention and early detection. Chapter 2 describes foundational information about genomics and germline testing. Important terms appear in bold throughout the book and are defined in the Glossary.

Nurses may face questions from patients about what occurs during a consultation with a genetics professional. Patients often want to know why the test cannot just be ordered. Genetic counseling involves multiple steps, including construction and interpretation of family pedigrees, ordering of tests, and interpretation of test results, all of which may have specific challenges. Nurses must be informed on the process so that they can reassure their patients that these steps are necessary. Chapter 3 provides an overview of the genetic counseling and testing process.

The increased awareness and direct-to-consumer marketing messages about genetic testing have prompted patients to ask more questions about genetic testing. Nurses must be able to respond to basic questions about different types of genomic testing with accurate information. If patients are concerned that healthcare professionals are not paying attention to their family history, they may turn to direct-to-consumer genetic testing, which may or may not provide the information they are seeking. Direct-to-consumer genetic testing is discussed in Chapter 4.

Following genetic testing, most genetics professionals provide detailed information about recommendations for care, including recommendations for ongoing prevention and early detection. For patients who are found to have a harmful pathogenic variant (historically known as a *mutation*), these recommendations can be extensive and are based on the personal and family medical history, as well as the specific pathogenic variant. Chapter 5 provides quick overviews of many of the more common germline pathogenic variants. These overviews include information on risks associated with each variant, recommendations for cancer prevention and early detection, and when to offer genetic testing. Each overview also includes reputable resources for more information.

With public awareness of genetic testing growing, nurses need a resource that provides them with more intensive information on germline cancer risk than they would typically receive during undergraduate or graduate education. This handbook provides nurses with the essentials to understand genomic and hereditary cancer risk, to assist in facilitating interprofessional care with genetics and other oncology professionals, and to provide their patients with accurate and reassuring information.

CHAPTER 1

Why Nurses Need to Integrate Genomics Into Oncology Care

INTRODUCTION

When people think about genetics and cancer care, they often think about hereditary risk for developing cancer. For oncology nurses, understanding how **genetics** and **genomics** affect cancer care is important because determining hereditary risk is a critical aspect of cancer care, as is understanding how genetic characteristics of the tumor influence cancer treatment decisions. Knowing when to refer patients for germline testing of hereditary cancer risk can be a challenge for oncology nurses.

Genomics is defined as the study of all of an individual's genes (the *genome*) and how genes function. The principal difference between *genomics* and *genetics* is that *genetics* scrutinizes the functioning and composition of the single **gene**, whereas *genomics* addresses all genes and their interrelationships to identify their combined influence on the growth and development of the organism (National Cancer Institute, n.d.). Germline genetic testing for hereditary cancer risk is one form of genomic testing. Genetic testing in a tumor can identify **somatic** pathogenic variants in a tumor that drive tumor growth. Both germline pathogenic variants and somatic pathogenic variants in a tumor provide valuable information about the prevention, early detection, and treatment of malignancy. Collectively, these concepts are referred to as *precision medicine* (National Cancer Institute, n.d.).

PRECISION MEDICINE

Precision medicine (also referred to as *personalized medicine*) is an approach to patient care that enables the selection of preventive measures, diagnostic evaluations, and treatments that are most likely to help patients based on individual characteristics. An individual's underlying genomic makeup and the genomic characteristics of the disease guide care. Although precision medicine is not a new concept, recent advances in science and technology have accelerated this area of research in cancer care, especially related to genetics and genomics (Brant & Mayer, 2017). When an individual is diagnosed with cancer, knowledge of genomic alterations in the tumor, the genomic makeup of the individual, and how these genetic changes cause the cancer to grow and spread enable healthcare providers to select the optimal treatment. Thus, the goal of precision medicine in cancer care is to select a treatment type that is most likely to be effective based on the genomic makeup of the individual and the tumor.

HEREDITARY RISK OF DEVELOPING CANCER

Approximately 10% of people diagnosed with cancer have an inherited germline predisposition for developing one or more cancers (National Comprehensive Cancer Network, 2020). Identification of these inherited genomic pathogenic variants influences treatment, such as risk-reducing surgery, or may guide screening recommendations, which may be more intensive than those recommended for the general population. The identification of a pathogenic germline variant also has implications for other family members, who have the option to undergo testing to determine if they would benefit from more intensive preventive and early-detection measures.

Some families have multiple individuals with a history of malignancy, suggesting a hereditary risk beyond what would be expected by normal probability. Advances in genomic science and testing have made it possible to identify families at risk for developing malignancies because of altered (mutated) harmful germline pathogenic variants in a gene. For some of these families, the risk of developing cancer can be as high as 80%–90% in a lifetime (National Comprehensive Cancer Network, 2020).

Germline testing is an evolving science, with new pathogenic variants frequently being identified and many more yet to be discovered. As a result, germline testing remains imperfect, and it is far from a certainty that a **pathogenic variant** (historically referred to as a **mutation**) will be discovered during testing. However, when germline testing does identify a pathogenic variant in a family, other family members who do not have a cancer diagnosis may be tested to clarify whether they are at higher risk for developing malignancy. If family members test positive for a pathogenic variant that confers a high risk of developing malignancy, healthcare providers can tailor recommendations to prevent cancer or to detect cancer in its early stages. Conversely, for those family members who test negative for a known pathogenic variant, aggressive screening or preventive surgery may not be needed. In these cases, it is usually appropriate to follow recommendations standard for the general population, after considering both maternal and paternal family history. Similarly, for families in which a pathogenic variant is not detected but the history is still suggestive of hereditary risk, healthcare providers should offer recommendations for prevention and early detection based on the personal risk factors and family history.

Famously, actress Angelina Jolie's decision in 2013 to have risk-reducing mastectomies and later bilateral salpingo-oophorectomies (removal of the fallopian tubes and ovaries) because of known hereditary cancer risk heightened public awareness to the availability and power of genetic testing. Her case also demonstrated that individuals could exert some control, albeit with significant surgeries, to reduce their risk of developing cancer (Baildam, 2019).

IMPLICATIONS FOR NURSES

Germline genetic testing is a powerful tool that carries the possibility of enabling individuals and their families to identify potential increased risk of developing cancer. Genetic testing for hereditary risk has moved far beyond testing exclusively for alterations in the *BRCA1* and *BRCA2* genes (Thomas et al., 2019). In fact, many **hereditary cancer syndromes** are associated with known pathogenic variants.

Nurses need fundamental knowledge of genomic science to be able to identify families who might have hereditary cancer risk and refer them for appropriate evaluation. Many families may not realize that they have potential risk, and nurses can correct common misconceptions. Understanding concepts in genomic science also enables nurses as patient educators to reinforce information about hereditary predisposition for developing cancer, as well as how genetic testing can guide recommendations for care not only for a patient but for other family members, as well. Individuals and families need ongoing psychosocial support to cope with the information and recommendations for care. Awareness of the complexity and diversity of potential germline genetic testing results enables nurses to provide support and ensure that recommendations for care are implemented.

SUMMARY

Genomic science is driving cancer care and offers opportunities to truly prevent cancer and to detect cancer early, as well as to select the best possible treatment through germline genetic testing. Identification of hereditary risk in one family member allows other family members to clarify their risk and implement appropriate recommendations for cancer prevention and early detection. This valuable information can ultimately decrease the morbidity and mortality associated with cancer and decrease the costs associated with cancer care by targeting those individuals who are most likely to benefit from intensive cancer prevention and early-detection measures.

REFERENCES

Baildam, A.D. (2019). Current knowledge of risk reducing mastectomy: Indications, techniques, results, benefits, harms. *Breast, 46,* 48–51. https://doi.org/10.1016/j.breast.2019.03.011

Brant, J.M., & Mayer, D.K. (2017). Precision medicine: Accelerating the science to revolutionize cancer care. *Clinical Journal of Oncology Nursing, 21*(6), 722–729. https://doi.org/10.1188/17.CJON.722-729

National Cancer Institute. (n.d.). *NCI dictionary of cancer terms.* https://www.cancer.gov/publications/dictionaries/cancer-terms

National Comprehensive Cancer Network. (2020). *NCCN Clinical Practice Guidelines in Oncology (NCCN Guidelines®): Genetic/familial high-risk assessment: Breast, ovarian, and pancreatic* [v.2.2021]. https://www.nccn.org/professionals/physician_gls/pdf/genetics_bop.pdf

Thomas, M.H., Higgs, L.K., Modesitt, S.C., Schroen, A.T., Ring, K.L., & Dillon, P.M. (2019). Cases and evidence for panel testing in cancer genetics: Is site-specific testing dead? *Journal of Genetic Counseling, 28*(3), 700–707. https://doi.org/10.1002/jgc4.1044

CHAPTER 2

Genomic Basis of Cancer

INTRODUCTION

In order to provide excellent genomic care, nurses must have a basic understanding of DNA function, genomic terms, and pedigree construction. This knowledge base enables nurses to provide education about basic genomic concepts to patients and families.

DNA AND GENOMICS

Deoxyribonucleic acid (DNA) is the hereditary material found in all organisms. The vast majority of DNA in humans is found in the nucleus of the cell and is referred to as *nuclear DNA*. Nuclear DNA is inherited from both parents. A small amount of DNA also exists in cells' mitochondria and is referred to as *mitochondrial DNA*, which is only inherited from the mother. The information contained in DNA is stored as a code made up of four chemical bases (nucleotides): adenine (A), guanine (G), cytosine (C), and thymine (T). Human DNA consists of approximately three billion bases, with the order of these bases varying by 1% across all humans (Gunder McClary, 2020). The order of these chemical bases determines the information available for building and maintaining a human being. A group of three bases in a row along a DNA strand codes to make 1 of 20 amino acids in the human body. Groups of amino acids are combined to create a protein. If a change in a base occurs, it may change the amino acid and possibly create a protein that does not function properly. Changes in the order of these bases can result in a harmful alteration leading to development of a disease, such as a malignancy (see Figure 2-1).

Genes are made up of DNA that provides the instructions for healthy cell growth and development. A pathogenic variant (historically referred to as a *mutation*) is an error in the DNA of a gene that prevents the gene from functioning correctly (Gunder McClary, 2020). Most malignancies are a result of somatic (acquired) pathogenic changes that occur after conception because of exposure

FIGURE 2-1 ▪ BASE PAIRS CODE FOR PROTEINS

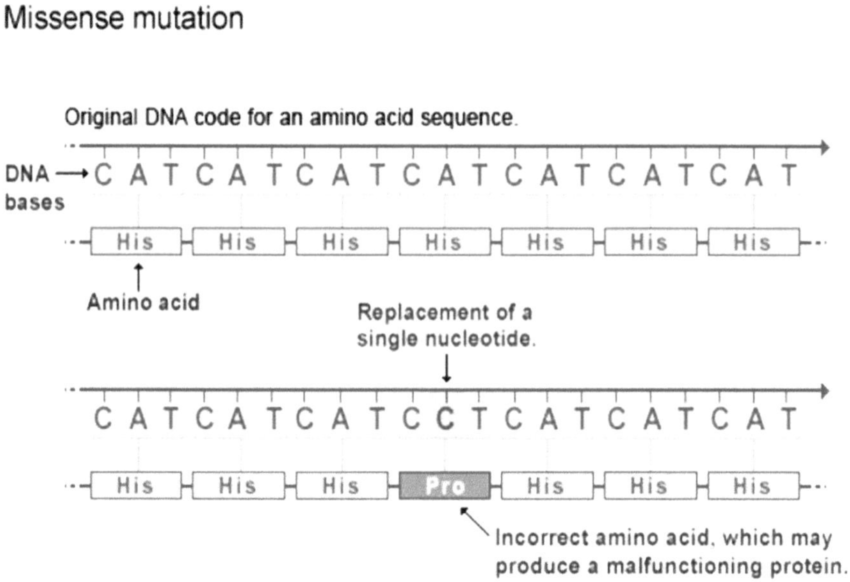

A change in a single base pair can result in a different or malfunctioning protein leading to disordered cell division and ultimately a malignancy.

Note. Image courtesy of U.S. National Library of Medicine (https://medlineplus.gov/genetics/understanding/mutationsanddisorders/possiblemutations).

to carcinogens. Somatic pathogenic changes occur in one cell and are passed on to new cells that arise from mitosis of the altered cell (Gunder McClary, 2020). These changes cannot be passed on to offspring because they were acquired after conception. Somatic pathogenic variants, also referred to as *sporadic*, can trigger a cell to become malignant and account for approximately 90% of cancers.

In some cases, germ cells (egg and sperm) carry a pathogenic change. After the egg is fertilized by the sperm, it becomes a single cell known as a **zygote**, which then divides many times to create a human being. Because all cells in the body originate from this first cell, the pathogenic variant is present in every cell in the body and can be passed on to the next generation (Gunder McClary, 2020). These germline pathogenic variants account for approximately 10% of cancers.

Humans have 23 pairs of **chromosomes** (46 chromosomes in total), which contain thousands of genes (see Figure 2-2). Each human also has two copies of every gene, with one copy from each parent. Most genetic changes that cause a hereditary form of cancer are inherited as an autosomal dominant disease and can be transmitted by only one parent. If an individual inherits an altered gene from one parent, every cell in the body is affected with the altered gene. Once the unaltered copy of the gene (from the other parent) in a cell becomes damaged from the environment or other exposure, malignant cells begin to proliferate. Because people with a hereditary cancer syndrome have an altered copy of the gene in every cell, they typically develop cancers more often than expected by chance and often at an early age (Gunder McClary, 2020).

Alleles are forms of the same gene with small differences in their sequence of **DNA bases**. Some of these differences are harmful, but most are harmless. Genetic alterations or changes that occur in more than 1% of the population are known as **polymorphisms** (Gunder McClary, 2020). These are common enough to be considered a harmless variation in the DNA and are responsible for human variation, such as eye or hair color.

The chance of passing on a pathogenic variant to an offspring applies equally to each pregnancy, as each parent provides one copy of each gene. If each parent contributes an unaltered working copy, the resulting offspring then has an average risk of developing cancer. If both copies are the same, it is considered **homozygous**. If the person has one altered and one unaltered copy, they are considered **heterozygous** for the condition. In autosomal dominant transmission, one altered copy can place the individual at increased risk for developing cancer. If a person has an autosomal dominant condition, there is a 50% chance of passing the altered copy to any offspring, whether male or female. This assumes that one parent has two unaltered copies (homozygous) and that the affected parent has one altered and one unaltered copy (heterozygous). The siblings of an individual with a pathogenic variant also have a 50% chance of having the same pathogenic variant if they share the same parent who carries the pathogenic variant.

FIGURE 2-2 ▪ GENES ARE CONTAINED IN CHROMOSOME

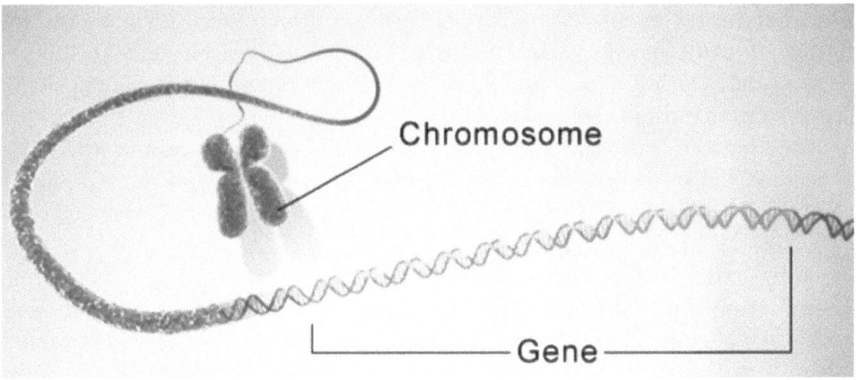

Each of the 46 chromosomes (23 pairs) have hundreds of genes.

Note. Image courtesy of U.S. National Library of Medicine (https://medlineplus.gov/genetics/understanding/basics/gene).

At conception, there is a 50% chance the parent will give the altered copy and a 50% chance the parent will give the unaltered working copy (Gunder McClary, 2020). The risk for other family members carrying the same pathogenic variant depends on how closely they are related to an affected individual.

In autosomal recessive transmission, two unaffected people must each carry one copy of the altered gene in order for offspring to be affected by the condition. If the offspring inherits two altered copies, they are considered homozygous for the condition and will be affected. Offspring of two carriers have a 25% chance of being affected by the disorder. With two carriers, each pregnancy has a 25% chance of producing a child who is affected, a 50% chance of producing a carrier of the gene, and a 25% chance of producing a child who is unaffected and not a carrier of the gene (Gunder McClary, 2020). Autosomal recessive hereditary cancer syndromes are much less common than autosomal dominant syndromes. Cancer risk is elevated in people who are homozygous with two altered copies.

Once a genetics professional has detected a pathogenic variant in a family, it is possible to calculate the statistical risk for other family members of carrying the same pathogenic variant, based on the principles of autosomal dominant and autosomal recessive transmission (Gunder McClary, 2020). In the case of autosomal dominance, first-degree relatives (children, siblings, and parents) have a 50% chance of having inherited the altered gene. Second-degree relatives (grandparents, aunts, and uncles) have a 25% chance of having the pathogenic variant.

NOMENCLATURE

Genetic testing reports are filled with specific information about the altered genes of interest. This is presented in a specific order and jargon referred to as **nomenclature**. Genetic testing reports provide information in nomenclature format about the specific variant and where it is located on the gene. This information about location is a combination of numbers and letters. This genetic "address" is made up of several parts.

The first piece of information in the address is the chromosome where the gene is located, represented by a number or letter. Chromosomes 1–22 (the autosomes) are designated by number, and the sex chromosomes are designated by X or Y (Gunder McClary, 2020).

Represented next is the arm of the chromosome where the gene is located. Each chromosome is divided into two sections, or arms, based on the location of a narrowing known as the *centromere*. By convention, the shorter arm is named *p*, and the longer arm is named *q* (Gunder McClary, 2020). For example, 6q is the long arm of chromosome 6.

The final piece of the address is the position of a gene based on a distinctive pattern of light and dark bands that appear when the chromosome is stained.

The number indicating the gene position increases with distance from the centromere. For example, 15q21 represents position 21 on the long arm of chromosome 15. In this case, 15q21 is closer to the centromere than 15q22.

The *CHEK2* gene is located at 22q12.1, which means it is located on the long (q) arm of chromosome 22 at position 12.1. More commonly on germline testing reports, the report will list the name of the gene, followed by the *c* for coding DNA sequence and the *p* for protein change (Haga et al., 2014). The affected gene, as well as the *c* and *p* data, are required when ordering testing for a relative when a family has a known pathogenic variant (see Figure 2-3).

FIGURE 2-3 ▪ COMPONENTS OF GENE NOMENCLATURE FOR *CHEK2* C.1100DELC (P.THR367METFS)

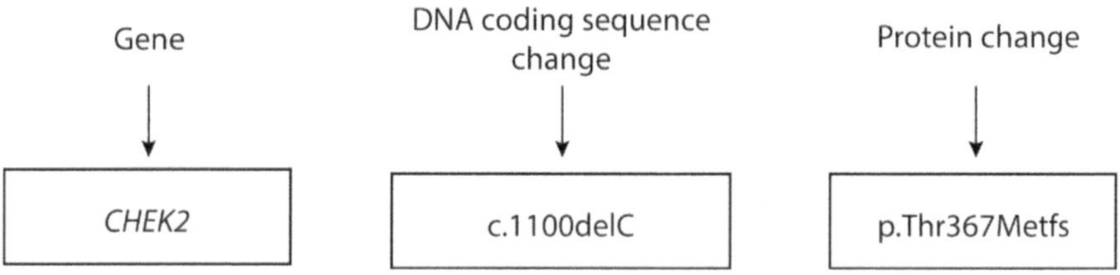

TERMS ENCOUNTERED IN GENOMIC CARE

Penetrance

Penetrance refers to the proportion of people with a specific pathogenic variant who exhibit signs and symptoms of the genetic syndrome. Different variants have different penetrance. For example, women with *BRCA1* or *BRCA2* pathogenic variants have up to a 41%–90% risk of developing breast cancer, and women with *ATM* pathogenic variants have an approximate 38% risk of developing breast cancer (National Comprehensive Cancer Network [NCCN], 2020a). *BRCA1* and *BRCA2* pathogenic variants are considered high-penetrance variants and *ATM* pathogenic variants are considered moderate-risk variants. Most pathogenic variants are associated with incomplete penetrance, meaning that not everyone who has the pathogenic variant will develop the malignancy in the case of hereditary cancer syndromes (Gunder McClary, 2020). Incomplete penetrance most likely results from a combination of genetic, environmental, and lifestyle factors, many of which are unknown. This phenomenon makes it challenging to predict whether or not cancer will develop, regardless of a pathogenic variant being passed on through different generations.

Variable Expressivity

Variable expressivity refers to the range of malignancies or symptoms that can occur in different people with the same genetic alteration (Gunder McClary, 2020). For example, in a family with a *BRCA1* pathogenic variant (commonly associated with breast and ovarian cancers), a range of outcomes can occur, including no cases of ovarian cancer, cases primarily of ovarian cancer, and a mix of cases of breast and ovarian cancer. Another example of variable expression can occur with a pathogenic variant in the *NF1* gene. One person may express a variant with café-au-lait macules, and another person might experience neurofibromas, breast cancer before age 50 years, or brain tumors (Friedman, 2019). As with incomplete penetrance, variable expressivity is most likely the result of a multiple genetic, environmental, and lifestyle factors, most of which have not been identified.

Mosaicism

Somatic pathogenic variants that occur in a single cell early in embryonic development can lead to a change known as **mosaicism** (Waldman & Mahon, 2017) (see Figure 2-4). These genetic changes are not present in a parent's egg or sperm cells or in the fertilized egg, but they occur later when the embryo has

FIGURE 2-4 ▪ PRESENTATION OF MOSAICISM CAUSED BY POSTZYGOTIC PATHOGENIC VARIANT

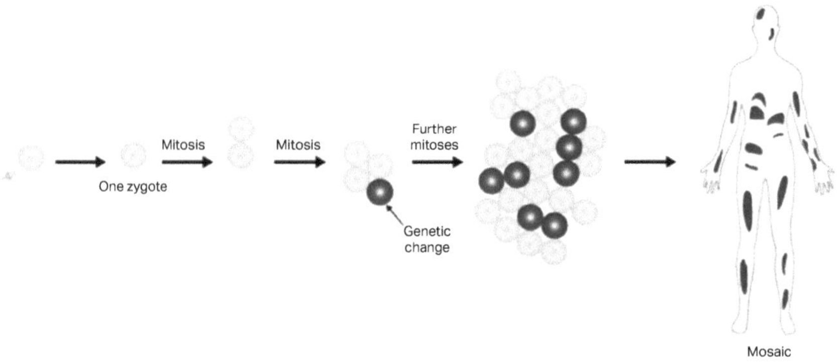

The egg and sperm join to form the zygote. After cell division, a genetic mutation occurs. The genetic change is present in some but not all cell lines. The earlier the mutation occurs, the more cell lines that are affected and the more likely the genetic change is to be expressed.

Note. Image courtesy of Genomics Education Programme (https://www.flickr.com/photos/genomicseducation/13080775333). Licensed under Attribution 2.0 Generic (CC BY 2.0; https://creativecommons.org/by/2.0).

expanded into several cells. As all the cells divide during growth and development, cells arising from the cell with the altered gene will contain the pathogenic variant, and other cells will not. Depending on the pathogenic variant and how many cells are affected, mosaicism may or may not cause health problems.

Founder Effect

Some genetic disorders are more likely to occur among people who trace their ancestry to a specific geographic area, which is referred to as the **founder effect**. Similarly, people in an ethnic group often share certain versions of their genes, which have been passed from common ancestors. If one of these shared genes contains a pathogenic variant, a particular hereditary syndrome may be seen more frequently in the group (Rebbeck et al., 2018). For example, 1 in 40 people of Ashkenazi Jewish ancestry carries one of three specific pathogenic variants in the *BRCA1* and *BRCA2* genes.

INDICATORS OF HEREDITARY RISK FOR DEVELOPING CANCER

Clinical Indicators of Hereditary Risk

The American College of Medical Genetics and Genomics, NCCN, and National Society of Genetic Counselors have compiled extensive resources that outline conditions in which patients and families should be referred for genetic testing (Hampel et al., 2015; Manahan et al., 2019; NCCN, 2020a). Figure 2-5 lists key indicators of hereditary risk to develop cancer.

Pedigree Construction

Every family has a starting point for initiating a genetic evaluation. A family member may be concerned about hereditary risk, or a person recently diagnosed with a malignancy may be considering treatment options. This person is referred to as the **proband**. The proband may or may not be diagnosed with cancer but frequently serves as a point of reference when discussing risk. In a three-generation pedigree, the proband is represented by an arrow in the figure (Mahon, 2016b).

A **pedigree** visually illustrates the relationship between family members and represents the transmission of a genetic trait across multiple generations in a family. A complete pedigree includes information about all relatives—maternal and paternal—including children, siblings, parents, aunts, uncles, cousins, and grandparents. Figure 2-6 represents the key components of pedigree construction and what should be included in every pedigree. The pedigree includes

FIGURE 2-5 ▪ KEY INDICATORS OF HEREDITARY RISK

- Characteristics in the patient
  - Cancer occurring at a younger age than expected in the general population, such as breast, endometrial, or colon cancer at age 50 years or younger
  - More than one primary cancer in one person, such as breast and ovarian cancer, or bilateral cancer in a paired organ, such as breast cancer in both breasts
  - Presence of premalignant conditions, such as 20 colorectal adenomatous polyps or dysplastic nevi
  - Cancer associated with hereditary risk, such as male breast cancer, ovarian cancer, retinoblastoma, pancreatic cancer, medullary thyroid cancer, paraganglioma, or a pheochromocytoma
- Characteristics in the family history
  - Evidence of autosomal dominant inheritance, such as two or more generations affected, with both men and women affected
  - Any pattern of cancer associated with a known cancer syndrome, such as breast, ovarian, endometrial, colon, or pancreatic cancer
  - Family history of rare cancers, such as ovarian cancer, male breast cancer, or pheochromocytoma
  - Known pathogenic variant in the family associated with an increased risk for developing cancer
- Characteristics in the tumor
  - **Microsatellite instability** in colon or endometrial cancer
  - **Triple-negative breast cancer** (i.e., estrogen receptor negative, progesterone receptor negative, HER2 not amplified) especially in a woman younger than age 60 years
  - **Gleason score** greater than 7 in prostate cancer
  - Higher allele count on tumor (somatic) testing

Note. Based on information from Forman & Sotelo, 2020; Hampel et al., 2015; National Comprehensive Cancer Network, 2020b.

a key identifying those cancer diagnoses, with diagnoses verified, if possible, by pathology reports or death certificates. Pedigrees should go beyond those affected by malignancy to include nonaffected family members. Age at the time of each cancer diagnosis is also recorded. Even if the cancer only appears to have occurred on one side of the family, a pedigree should still include both maternal and paternal sides. Ancestry is also recorded to identify individuals and family members who might have additional risk related to ethnicity. See Figure 2-7 for an example pedigree that is suggestive of hereditary risk. Pedigrees should be updated annually, with the diagnosis of cancer, when family history changes, when genetic testing occurs, and when results become available (Mahon, 2016b).

The manner in which pedigree information is extracted has a direct effect on the accuracy of the pedigree, which ultimately influences recommendations for cancer prevention and early detection. Asking a general question such as, "Has anyone in your family been diagnosed with cancer?" will typically yield much less information than if the healthcare provider systematically asks about each relative and methodically records the information.

FIGURE 2-6 ▪ KEY COMPONENTS INCLUDED IN PEDIGREE CONSTRUCTION

- Proband, offspring, parents, and maternal and paternal grandparents, aunts, uncles, and first cousins
- Age of all family members or age at death
- Indication of whether the individual is living or deceased: If deceased, include the cause of death.
- Affected status to identify who in the family has a diagnosis of cancer, including age at diagnosis
- For multiple cancers, different shading or colors to indicate each cancer or disease (key included)
- Adoption status, if applicable
- **Consanguinity** (parents or other close relatives are related)
- Ethnicity of each grandparent (e.g., German, Native American, Polish, African American)
- Date pedigree was obtained or revised

FIGURE 2-7 ▪ PEDIGREE SUGGESTIVE OF HEREDITARY RISK

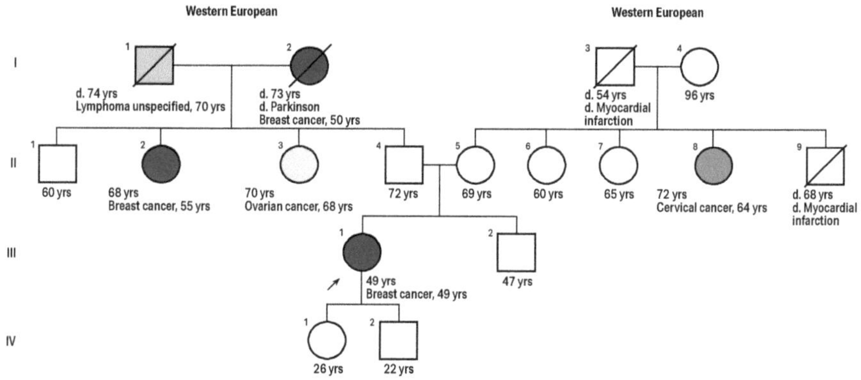

Interpreting a Pedigree

The Roman numerals represent generations. The pedigree in this example has four generations. Genetics professionals always attempt to construct at least a three-generation pedigree. The Arabic numerals represent individuals within a generation. Squares represent males, and circles represent females. A slash represents a deceased person, and filled-in circles and squares represent diagnoses confirmed with pathology reports. The current age or age at death is documented for each person. In cancer-related genetic evaluations, cancer diagnoses are documented with age at onset and, if possible, other aspects of the tumor (e.g., hormone receptors). If a genetic pathogenic variant is identified in a family, that information can be added.

During pedigree construction, sensitive and inclusive language regarding biologic sex and gender identification is important. The pedigree should reflect biologic sex at birth in order to provide appropriate recommendations for care, and the rationale for this inclusion should be communicated to a patient in a sensitive way, using the individual's self-identified pronouns (Hales, 2020). For example, a person may identify as male but was assigned female at birth. If this individual is found to have a pathogenic variant in *BRCA2* and still has ovaries or breast tissue, he may want to consider risk-reducing surgery.

In 1995, the National Society of Genetic Counselors published standardized criteria for the graphic presentation of data in pedigrees; these remain the current standard for pedigree construction (Bennett et al., 2008). Pedigrees can be constructed with pencil and paper and scanned into a patient's medical record; however, most genetics professionals utilize pedigree software to construct the pedigree, making the process of updating the pedigree more efficient as more pertinent information becomes available.

Barriers to Constructing an Effective Pedigree

A number of barriers can affect the construction and utilization of pedigrees. Family communication and dynamics may limit the availability and the accuracy of the information. In addition to time constraints in busy oncology practices, other barriers may impede pedigree construction (see Table 2-1). Nurses need to be aware of these barriers and take direct action to reduce or eliminate them whenever possible.

Adoption presents significant challenges to pedigree construction. Some individuals have no knowledge of the biologic health of one or both parents, or they may not want to or cannot locate their biologic parents to obtain this information. Some individuals who are adopted or have limited knowledge of their biologic family may be more successful than others in obtaining health information. This issue can be distressing for some individuals and must be approached in a sensitive way.

LABORATORY CONSIDERATIONS

Types of Testing

The type of testing offered depends on the pedigree, personal history of the patient, and prior testing in the family. If the pedigree suggests the possibility of several germline predisposition syndromes, testing will typically begin with a panel of multiple genes associated with cancers. If a pathogenic variant is detected, other family members can undergo targeted single-site variant testing.

TABLE 2-1 ▪ BARRIERS TO THE IMPLEMENTATION OF QUALITY PEDIGREES

Barrier	Possible Remedy
Patient Factors	
Inaccurate family history	Try to verify diagnoses with pathology reports, prior testing reports, or death certificates.
Lack of desire to explore family history	Educate the patient about why an accurate family history is important to constructing an accurate risk assessment and possibly ordering and interpreting genetic testing results.
Limited family history	Encourage the patient to reach out to other relatives prior to the appointment to try to obtain as much information as possible.
Patient adopted	No remedy: Explain to the patient that risk assessment is difficult and that the interpretation of genetic testing results may be limited or noninformative.
Small family structure	No remedy: Explain to the patient that this may limit the accuracy of the information.
Unknown paternity	No remedy: Explain to the patient that risk assessment is difficult and that the interpretation of genetic testing results may be limited or noninformative.
Provider Factors	
Failure to recognize subtle indicators of hereditary risk	Provide ongoing continuing information about emerging genetic syndromes.
Time required to construct pedigree	Have the patient gather some of the information prior to the visit, and document the information on paper or directly into a computer program.
System Factors	
No inclusion of decision support and red flags for referral to genetics professional in electronic health record	Users should identify criteria that must be collected and help to develop an interface that provides clinical decision-making support.
No reimbursement for time to collect accurate pedigree	Users need to lobby for changes in reimbursement that acknowledge the benefits of a comprehensive, accurate three-generation pedigree.
No visual representation in electronic health record	Users should provide feedback to develop appropriate family history sections with a usable family history interface and produce a visual pedigree with standard symbols.

Note. Based on information from Armel et al., 2009; Beadles et al., 2014; Lu et al., 2014; Riley et al., 2012; Venne & Scheuner, 2015; Wood et al., 2014; Ziogas & Anton-Culver, 2003.

From "The Three-Generation Pedigree: A Critical Tool in Cancer Genetics Care" by S.M. Mahon, 2016b, *Oncology Nursing Forum, 43*(5), p. 659, https://doi.org/10.1188/16.ONF.655-660. Copyright 2016 by Oncology Nursing Society. Reprinted with permission.

Historically, testing for germline hereditary predisposition syndromes utilized the **Sanger DNA sequencing** method that tests for one or two genes (Smith, 2019). Just as a spell-check program looks for a punctuation or typographical error by reading an entire paragraph, sequencing can identify when a base pair is added or deleted and when the wrong base pair is substituted or inserted. Sanger sequencing can only analyze and determine the nucleotide sequence of short pieces of DNA and is very time-consuming. Usually, this methodology is limited to approximately 300–1,000 base pairs. The quality of a Sanger sequence is often inaccurate in the first 15–40 bases because that is where the primer binds. However, it is valuable for confirming that a specific alteration is present or absent and is also useful in targeted single-site testing or confirming a pathogenic variant following larger panel testing.

In contrast to Sanger sequencing, the introduction of **next-generation sequencing** (NGS) offers a different form of genetic testing technology that allows multiple genes to be analyzed simultaneously and much more quickly through an automated process (Price et al., 2018). This has led to the development of tests that incorporate panels of genes to analyze less common cancer susceptibility genes. NGS has led to reduced cost and turnaround time in genetic testing.

Many hereditary cancer syndromes have confusing clinical presentations, and it can be challenging to select the appropriate test. Simultaneous testing for germline pathogenic variants with a panel of genes associated with multiple hereditary cancer syndromes using an NGS-targeted platform may be more efficient and cost effective. NGS has made the detection of more pathogenic variants possible, especially in less common genes. However, it has greatly increased the complexity of genetic counseling, the genetic testing process, and the interpretation of test results (Stanislaw et al., 2016). Although NGS has become the standard in panels of genes associated with hereditary predisposition to developing cancer, Sanger sequencing is still used in laboratories, primarily for some single-gene sequencing, for single-site testing of known familial pathogenic variants, and for confirmatory purposes following NGS analysis (Smith, 2019).

Single-nucleotide polymorphism (SNP) genotyping is another type of genetic testing methodology. This type of test checks for the presence or absence of specific variants throughout the genetic code, such as particular SNPs or small insertions or deletions. SNPs are genetic variations that represent a difference in a single nucleotide in the DNA (Price et al., 2018). SNP genotyping only looks at pieces of DNA, which is much different than sequencing an entire gene by examining the entire sequence of nucleotides. This technology is commonly utilized in direct-to-consumer genetic testing (Mahon, 2016a).

Accuracy of Testing

Another consideration in genomic care is whether the genetic test is valid and useful. A genetic test is valid if it provides an accurate result. Two main measures of accuracy apply to genetic tests: analytical validity and clinical validity. A genetic test's usefulness refers to clinical utility.

Analytical validity refers to how well the test predicts the presence or absence of a specific genetic alteration (Price et al., 2018). Can the test accurately detect whether a specific genetic variant is present or absent?

Clinical validity refers to how well the genetic variant being analyzed is related to the presence, absence, or risk of a specific disease (Lee et al., 2019). For example, is a gene on a particular panel truly associated with an increased risk for developing a specific cancer? NCCN (2020a) notes that many of the genes on hereditary breast and ovarian cancer susceptibility panels have not been systematically examined to determine clinical validity and to understand the strength of association with developing these cancers.

Clinical utility refers to whether the test can provide information about diagnosis, treatment, management, or prevention of a disease that will be helpful to a patient. NCCN (2020a) notes that, similar to clinical validity, many of the genes on hereditary breast and ovarian cancer panels do not have specific medical management recommendations.

All laboratories that perform health-related testing, including genetic testing, must follow federal regulatory standards, known as the Clinical Laboratory Improvement Amendments (CLIA). CLIA standards cover how tests are performed, qualifications for laboratory personnel, and quality control and testing procedures for each laboratory. By controlling the quality of laboratory practices, CLIA standards are designed to ensure the analytical validity of genetic tests (U.S. Food and Drug Administration, 2020).

CLIA standards do not address the clinical validity or clinical utility of genetic tests (Stoffel & Carethers, 2020). The U.S. Food and Drug Administration requires information about clinical validity for some genetic tests. Additionally, the State of New York requires information on clinical validity for all laboratory tests performed for people living in that state. Consumers, healthcare providers, researchers, policy makers, and health insurance companies often determine the clinical utility of a genetic test (Farkas, 2016).

SUMMARY

All nurses, regardless of practice setting, need to understand basic concepts surrounding how germline pathogenic variants are transmitted, how they are detected, and how they affect oncology care. Identifying families with potential hereditary risk requires knowledge of the key indicators of hereditary risk and how to construct and interpret a complete and accurate pedigree. Families with potential germline risk should be referred to a credentialed genetics professional for evaluation. Nurses also must be able to answer basic questions about germline testing, including how it is processed, concepts of accuracy, and the utility of the testing. Patients and families look to nurses for information on these basic concepts and guidance on how to obtain accurate information and specialized care from a credentialed genetics professional.

REFERENCES

Armel, S.R., McCuaig, J., Finch, A., Demsky, R., Panzarella, T., Murphy, J., & Rosen, B. (2009). The effectiveness of family history questionnaires in cancer genetic counseling. *Journal of Genetic Counseling, 18*(4), 366–378. https://doi.org/10.1007/s10897-009-9228-x

Beadles, C.A., Ryanne Wu, R., Himmel, T., Buchanan, A.H., Powell, K.P., Hauser, E., ... Orlando, L.A. (2014). Providing patient education: Impact on quantity and quality of family health history collection. *Familial Cancer, 13*(2), 325–332. https://doi.org/10.1007/s10689-014-9701-z

Bennett, R.L., French, K.S., Resta, R.G., & Doyle, D.L. (2008). Standardized human pedigree nomenclature: Update and assessment of the recommendations of the National Society of Genetic Counselors. *Journal of Genetic Counseling, 17*(5), 424–433. https://doi.org/10.1007/s10897-008-9169-9

Farkas, D.H. (2016). Clinical validity and utility: Putting the patient front and center. *Journal of Molecular Diagnostics, 18*(5), 635–637. https://doi.org/10.1016/j.jmoldx.2016.06.003

Forman, A., & Sotelo, J. (2020). Tumor-based genetic testing and familial cancer risk. *Cold Spring Harbor Perspectives in Medicine, 10*(8), a036590. https://doi.org/10.1101/cshperspect.a036590

Friedman, J.M. (2019). Neurofibromatosis 1. In M.P. Adam, H.H. Ardinger, R.A. Pagon, & S.E. Wallace (Eds.), *GeneReviews®*. University of Washington. https://www.ncbi.nlm.nih.gov/books/NBK1109

Gunder McClary, L.M. (2020). *Essentials of medical genetics for nursing and health professionals: An interprofessional approach.* Jones and Bartlett Learning.

Haga, S.B., Mills, R., Pollak, K.I., Rehder, C., Buchanan, A.H., Lipkus, I.M., ... Datto, M. (2014). Developing patient-friendly genetic and genomic test reports: Formats to promote patient engagement and understanding. *Genome Medicine, 6*, 58. https://doi.org/10.1186/s13073-014-0058-6

Hales, K.G. (2020). Signaling inclusivity in undergraduate biology courses through deliberate framing of genetics topics relevant to gender identity, disability, and race. *CBE—Life Sciences Education, 19*(2), es2. https://doi.org/10.1187/cbe.19-08-0156

Hampel, H., Bennett, R.L., Buchanan, A., Pearlman, R., & Wiesner, G.L. (2015). A practice guideline from the American College of Medical Genetics and Genomics and the National Society of Genetic Counselors: Referral indications for cancer predisposition assessment. *Genetics in Medicine, 17*(1), 70–87. https://doi.org/10.1038/gim.2014.147

Lee, K., Seifert, B.A., Shimelis, H., Ghosh, R., Crowley, S.B., Carter, N.J., ... Couch, F.J. (2019). Clinical validity assessment of genes frequently tested on hereditary breast and ovarian cancer susceptibility sequencing panels. *Genetics in Medicine, 21*(7), 1497–1506. https://doi.org/10.1038/s41436-018-0361-5

Lu, K.H., Wood, M.E., Daniels, M., Burke, C., Ford, J., Kauff, N.D., ... Hughes, K.S. (2014). American Society of Clinical Oncology expert statement: Collection and use of a cancer family history for oncology providers. *Journal of Clinical Oncology, 32*(8), 833–840. https://doi.org/10.1200/jco.2013.50.9257

Mahon, S.M. (2016a). The deceptive appeal of direct-to-consumer genetics. *Annals of Internal Medicine, 165*(9), 675–676. https://doi.org/10.7326/L16-0333

Mahon, S.M. (2016b). The three-generation pedigree: A critical tool in cancer genetics care. *Oncology Nursing Forum, 43*(5), 655–660. https://doi.org/10.1188/16.ONF.655-660

Manahan, E.R., Kuerer, H.M., Sebastian, M., Hughes, K.S., Boughey, J.C., Euhus, D.M., ... Taylor, W.A. (2019). Consensus guidelines on genetic testing for hereditary breast cancer from the American Society of Breast Surgeons. *Annals of Surgical Oncology, 26*(10), 3025–3031. https://doi.org/10.1245/s10434-019-07549-8

National Comprehensive Cancer Network. (2020a). *NCCN Clinical Practice Guidelines in Oncology (NCCN Guidelines®): Genetic/familial high-risk assessment: Breast, ovarian, and pancreatic* [v.2.2021]. https://www.nccn.org/professionals/physician_gls/pdf/genetics_bop.pdf

National Comprehensive Cancer Network. (2020b). *NCCN Clinical Practice Guidelines in Oncology (NCCN Guidelines®): Genetic/familial high-risk assessment: Colorectal* [v.1.2020]. https://www.nccn.org/professionals/physician_gls/pdf/genetics_colon.pdf

Price, K.S., Svenson, A., King, E., Ready, K., & Lazarin, G.A. (2018). Inherited cancer in the age of next-generation sequencing. *Biological Research for Nursing, 20*(2), 192–204. https://doi.org/10.1177/1099800417750746

Rebbeck, T.R., Friebel, T.M., Friedman, E., Hamann, U., Huo, D., Kwong, A., ... Nathanson, K.L. (2018). Mutational spectrum in a worldwide study of 29,700 families with *BRCA1* or *BRCA2* mutations. *Human Mutation, 39*(5), 593–620. https://doi.org/10.1002/humu.23406

Riley, B.D., Culver, J.O., Skrzynia, C., Senter, L.A., Peters, J.A., Costalas, J.W., ... Trepanier, A.M. (2012). Essential elements of genetic cancer risk assessment, counseling, and testing: Updated recommendations of the National Society of Genetic Counselors. *Journal of Genetic Counseling, 21*(2), 151–161. https://doi.org/10.1007/s10897-011-9462-x

Smith, L.P. (2019). The spectrum of genetic testing. *Seminars in Oncology Nursing, 35*(1), 11–21. https://doi.org/10.1016/j.soncn.2018.12.008

Stanislaw, C., Xue, Y., & Wilcox, W.R. (2016). Genetic evaluation and testing for hereditary forms of cancer in the era of next-generation sequencing. *Cancer Biology and Medicine, 13*(1), 55–67. https://doi.org/10.28092/j.issn.2095-3941.2016.0002

Stoffel, E.M., & Carethers, J.M. (2020). Current approaches to germline cancer genetic testing. *Annual Review of Medicine, 71*(1), 85–102. https://doi.org/10.1146/annurev-med-052318-101009

U.S. Food and Drug Administration. (2020). Clinical Laboratory Improvement Amendments (CLIA). https://www.fda.gov/medical-devices/ivd-regulatory-assistance/clinical-laboratory-improvement-amendments-clia

Venne, V.L., & Scheuner, M.T. (2015). Securing and documenting cancer family history in the age of the electronic medical record. *Surgical Oncology Clinics of North America, 24*(4), 639–652. https://doi.org/10.1016/j.soc.2015.06.001

Waldman, L., & Mahon, S.M. (2017). Mosaicism: Implications for genetic counseling and medical management. *Clinical Journal of Oncology Nursing, 21*(4), 428–432. https://doi.org/10.1188/17.CJON.428-432

Wood, M.E., Kadlubek, P., Pham, T.H., Wollins, D.S., Lu, K.H., Weitzel, J.N., ... Hughes, K.S. (2014). Quality of cancer family history and referral for genetic counseling and testing among oncology practices: A pilot test of quality measures as part of the American Society of Clinical Oncology Quality Oncology Practice Initiative. *Journal of Clinical Oncology, 32*(8), 824–829. https://doi.org/10.1200/JCO.2013.51.4661

Ziogas, A., & Anton-Culver, H. (2003). Validation of family history data in cancer family registries. *American Journal of Preventive Medicine, 24*(2), 190–198. https://doi.org/10.1016/S0749-3797(02)00593-7

CHAPTER 3

Genomic Risk Assessment and Testing

INTRODUCTION

Many activities occur when an individual or family is referred to or seeks genetic counseling services with a credentialed genetics professional to better understand potential risk for developing cancer. All nurses must provide patients and families with basic information about what to expect during a genetic counseling appointment, to adequately prepare them and decrease anxiety about genetic testing. Understanding what happens during genetic counseling appointments and the rationale for these activities enables oncology nurses to educate patients on what to expect, how to prepare, and why the appointment is so important in comprehensive cancer care.

Many families are surprised to learn that an initial evaluation in a genetic counseling appointment lasts 60–90 minutes (Mahon, 2013). Genetic testing for germline cancer risk is much more complicated than looking for a few criteria and ordering a panel of tests (Morganti et al., 2019). Providing information on the potential strengths, limitations, and risks associated with testing; selecting the best person in which to initiate testing to obtain informative results; interpreting test results; providing recommendations for care; coordinating care for the entire family; and enrolling patients and families in research studies are important aspects of the genetic counseling process that are routinely implemented by genetics professionals (see Figure 3-1).

RISK ASSESSMENT

Genetic counseling and testing can be extremely helpful for some individuals and families to clarify cancer risk and, in some cases, for making treatment decisions. As patients prepare for a genetic counseling appointment, it is important that nurses instruct them on why they are being referred and that genetic coun-

FIGURE 3-1 ▪ GENETICS PROFESSIONALS

- Geneticists are physicians with board certification in genetics from the American Board of Medical Genetics and Genomics. They complete a fellowship in genetics and pass a board examination through the American Board of Medical Genetics and Genomics.
- Licensed genetic counselors are healthcare professionals with specialized graduate degrees in the areas of medical genetics and counseling. Currently, there are more than 30 accredited programs in genetic counseling in the United States. The American Board of Genetic Counseling certifies genetic counselors. The National Society of Genetic Counselors maintains a website (www.nsgc.org) that can provide healthcare professionals and the public with information on credentialed genetics professionals by zip code.
- Credentialed genetics nurses have specialized education and training in genetics. They can be certified by the American Nurses Credentialing Center with an Advanced Genetic Nurse-Board Certified (AGN-BC) credential or by the Nurse Portfolio Credentialing Commission and hold an Advanced Clinical Genetic Nurse (ACGN) or Clinical Genetic Nurse (CGN) credential.

seling can help them better understand their cancer risks and hereditary risks, which have implications for patients and family members. Nurses should stress that the purpose of the visit is for patient education and risk assessment, which may include genetic testing.

Nurses should also emphasize that a referral for evaluation of potential hereditary risk is not an order for genetic testing. The genetics professional may not recommend genetic testing. Patients must be made aware that pursuing genetic testing is their personal choice. Patients should understand that the purpose of the appointment is to provide them with the education necessary to make an informed decision that is best for the individual.

Individuals who have a family history of cancer often start by speaking with their primary care provider or oncologist about their cancer risk. The National Comprehensive Cancer Network (NCCN) and American Society of Clinical Oncology recommend regular risk assessment and referral for hereditary cancer syndrome assessment if a genetic risk is suspected, and the American College of Surgeons accreditation requires that genetics services be made available to patients (Lu et al., 2014; NCCN, 2020a). Patients and families might also inquire about risk or parameters for genetic testing.

At diagnosis of malignancy, patients and family members may have questions and concerns about hereditary predisposition, which they may or may not articulate (Shane-Carson & Jeter, 2019). This is often an excellent opportunity for a teachable moment about potential hereditary risk. Nurses can initiate the discussion by saying, "Family members are often worried about their risk when a loved one is diagnosed with cancer. This is a common reaction. Would you like to know more about this?"

At another point in the cancer care trajectory—the completion of definitive therapy when a survivorship care plan is implemented—patients may have concerns about hereditary risk or may be more open to exploring genetic testing (Boehm et al., 2019). This can be an opportunity to review if testing was performed or if a referral is appropriate.

A genetics professional can provide an individual with enough information for them to decide if testing is appropriate, who in the family to test, and what tests to order. Because genetic testing has implications for an individual and a family, many genetics professionals will provide education and counseling to multiple family members and, when possible, provide encouragement for family members to discuss testing.

If an individual or healthcare provider is concerned about hereditary risk, a credentialed genetics provider can help a patient understand risks and discuss if genetic testing would be useful. This can facilitate individualized recommendations for care based on assessment while helping an individual to understand the risk for developing cancer and how to best manage personal risk.

THE IMPORTANCE OF FAMILY MEDICAL HISTORY

The decision to offer genetic testing is based on a patient's personal medical history, personal risk factors for developing cancer, family history of cancer, and, if an individual has a cancer diagnosis, the characteristics of the tumor. All of these factors directly influence the selection of genetic tests or the panel of genes ordered. Understanding the family medical history also influences recommendations for screening and prevention. The accuracy of the family medical history plays a vital role in selecting these recommendations.

The first step in the cancer genetic counseling process is to gather information that will be needed for the risk assessment. Families may not be aware of the medical histories of relatives, especially those who are more distant in relation, such as aunts, uncles, or cousins. Prior to an appointment, most genetics professionals will ask family members to complete a form that details as much information as possible about the family medical history. This may require a patient to contact extended family members in order to gather the information. With the legwork out of the way, patients can arrive at the appointment with the family medical information that is necessary to proceed with the risk assessment. Patients may complete this assessment on paper and bring it to the appointment, or the assessment can be completed electronically through Health Insurance Portability and Accountability Act–compliant software that gathers the data and generates a pedigree that can be modified and edited as needed.

During the initial visit, the genetics professional will ask multiple questions about the health and medical history of family members and relatives, including a discussion of the health and lifestyle of children, siblings, parents, aunts, uncles, cousins, and grandparents. This step provides crucial information so the genetics professional can make the most accurate risk calculations and choose the appropriate genetic tests. In addition, the genetics professional will want to know which relatives are still living and their ages or, if deceased, their age at death and cause of death. The genetics professional will also collect information about any family member who has a cancer diagnosis, as well as premalignant conditions, such as colon polyps. Because some ethnic groups are at higher risk for hereditary cancers, the genetics professional will ask questions about ancestry. The genetics professional will utilize all this information to construct the pedigree and to calculate the risk of developing cancer and the risk of carrying a germline pathogenic variant.

DEVELOPING A PEDIGREE

As discussed in Chapter 2, a pedigree displays information about the family history in a visual format, making patterns of genetic transmission and possible genetic syndromes easier to identify. A pedigree can also be an excellent visual teaching tool to educate the family about genetic concepts. Most genetics professionals will provide the patient with a copy of the pedigree. The information in the pedigree also helps the genetics professional identify the best person or people in the family to initially test. If a test detects a pathogenic variant, the pedigree can be used to identify which other family members should be offered testing. Combined with genetic testing results, the pedigree provides extensive information so the genetics professional can make the best recommendations possible for cancer prevention and detection.

The pedigree should be reviewed at least annually and updated any time family history changes, or as the results of genetic testing become available for family members (Mahon, 2016). In some families, pedigree information is incomplete, which limits its accuracy. In some cases, family members are estranged, or an individual does not have contact with an entire side of the family. Individuals who were adopted may have limited or no information about their genetic family history. The genetics professional will discuss how these problems affect genetic testing decisions and interpretation of results (Cleophat et al., 2018).

In general, a pedigree provides information about family medical history. Risk assessment also considers the medical and lifestyle history of the proband (the person who is the starting point or of interest for the genetic evaluation of a family). For women, this may include information about menstrual and pregnancy history and exogenous hormone use. Lifestyle factors that are considered include height, weight, diet, exercise, ultraviolet light exposure, tobacco use, vaccination history, and cancer screening history, such as mammography or colonoscopy. With lifestyle information being discussed, there is an opportunity to educate patients and families about the importance of a healthy lifestyle. An estimated 42% of cancer cases and 45% of cancer deaths in the United States are attributed to modifiable risk factors, such as diet, exercise, and tobacco use (American Cancer Society, 2019).

Once the pedigree is complete, the genetics professional evaluates the pedigree and considers personal medical history and risk factors. The genetics professional will discuss any increased risks for cancer. Sometimes, genetic testing is not recommended, but more vigilant screening might be an effective option. Often, some type of genetic testing will be recommended. The decision whether to undergo genetic testing is based on information in the pedigree, as well as personal risk factors.

RISK CALCULATIONS

The accuracy of the pedigree influences the accuracy of risk calculations and the selection of the most appropriate genetic tests. Although genetic testing results that show a pathogenic variant have a direct influence on recommendations for prevention and screening, risk calculations often have a direct influence for individuals and families who have suspected germline risk but no identified pathogenic variant. Software programs and models can calculate statistical risks for developing cancer, as well as the risk of having a pathogenic variant (Shane-Carson & Jeter, 2019) (see Figure 3-2).

As part of the genetic counseling process, the genetics professional reviews the incidence of cancer in the general population, comparing the incidence rates with the individual's personal calculated risk. Based on an individual's specific personal and family medical history, the individual's percentages could differ from the general population norm. For example, the average population risk of developing breast cancer is approximately 12%–13% (American Cancer Society, 2020).

The Tyrer-Cuzick model is used to calculate a person's likelihood of carrying a *BRCA1* or *BRCA2* pathogenic variant. This model also estimates the likelihood of a woman developing breast cancer in 10 years and during the course of her lifetime. For example, a 38-year-old woman with a mother diagnosed with premenopausal breast cancer at age 45 years and a maternal aunt diagnosed with postmenopausal breast cancer at age 63 years is found to have a greater lifetime risk of developing breast cancer. With this model, her lifetime risk is 26%, slightly more than double the average. In this example, knowing this information helps a patient understand the magnitude of her cancer risk based on family history. Because her risk is estimated to be greater than 20% based on the modeling, more intensive screening, including a possible breast magnetic resonance imaging (MRI) scan with mammography, is a consideration (NCCN, 2020a). Furthermore, if the woman is found to have a germline risk for devel-

FIGURE 3-2 ▪ TYPES OF MODELS UTILIZED IN RISK FACTOR ASSESSMENT

- Models to estimate breast cancer risk
  - The Claus model estimates breast cancer risk in 10-year increments in women without a diagnosis of breast cancer who have a family history of breast and/or ovarian cancer.
  - The Gail model estimates breast cancer risk in 5-year increments and lifetime risk in women age 35 years or older without a diagnosis of cancer who have a minimal to moderate family history of breast cancer. A known limitation is that it does not consider paternal history or ovarian cancer history.
  - The Tyrer-Cuzick model estimates risk of breast cancer in the next 10 years and over a lifetime. The model considers age, age at menarche, parity, age at first delivery, height and weight, and family history of breast and ovarian cancer on the maternal and paternal sides. The model considers if the woman has had genetic testing and if it was negative.
- Models to estimate risk of a *BRCA1* and/or *BRCA2* pathogenic variant
  - BRCAPro estimates the risk of carrying a *BRCA1* or *BRCA2* pathogenic variant in women with a personal and family history of breast and/or ovarian cancer.
  - The Penn II model estimates the risk of carrying *BRCA1* or *BRCA2* pathogenic variant in women with personal and family history of breast, ovarian, pancreatic, and/or prostate cancer.
  - The Tyrer-Cuzick model estimates the risk of carrying a *BRCA1* or *BRCA2* pathogenic variant in women with a family history of breast and/or ovarian cancer.
- Models to identify families at risk for hereditary colorectal cancer
  - The Amsterdam criteria identifies the presence of specific family history criteria suggestive of Lynch syndrome, which should lead to referral for genetic evaluation.
  - The Bethesda model identifies the presence of a cluster of defined criteria suggestive of Lynch syndrome, which should lead to referral for genetic evaluation.
  - The PREMM model estimates the risk of carrying a pathogenic variant associated with Lynch syndrome in people with a family history of colorectal and gynecologic cancer.

Note. Based on information from Hampel et al., 2015; National Comprehensive Cancer Network, 2020a, 2020b.

oping breast cancer, her risk may be substantially higher than 26%. A germline pathogenic variant is passed directly from a parent to a child at the time of conception. Hereditary predisposition accounts for approximately 10% of all cancer diagnoses. However, if a germline pathogenic variant is detected in the family and the woman tests negative for the known variant, her risk would likely be closer to that of a woman in the general population. Even if a pathogenic variant is not detected in the patient or a family member, her risk may still be elevated, and the risk modeling can be helpful in managing care and making recommendations for cancer prevention and early detection.

Risk modeling has distinct strengths and limitations (Cintolo-Gonzalez et al., 2017). If the family is small, these models can underestimate or overestimate the risk of having a pathogenic variant or developing cancer. To be most accurate, information about all relatives must be included, not only the people with a cancer diagnosis, to prevent overestimation of risk. For example, a 42-year-old woman was referred for evaluation of hereditary risk and discussion of risk-reducing surgery based on the following pedigree.

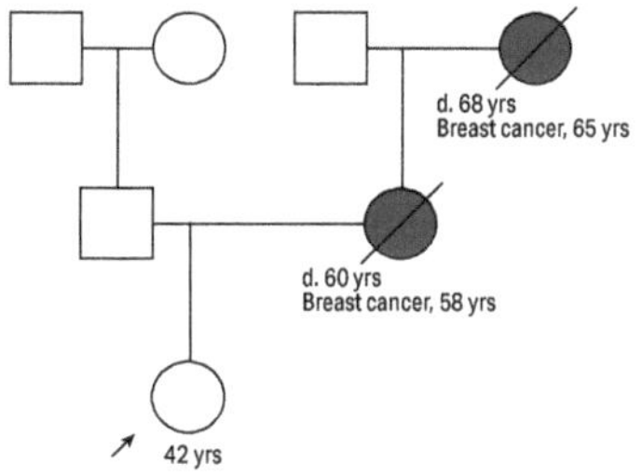

Her Tyrer-Cuzick lifetime risk of developing cancer is estimated to be 30%. However, a more inclusive pedigree provides a different risk calculation.

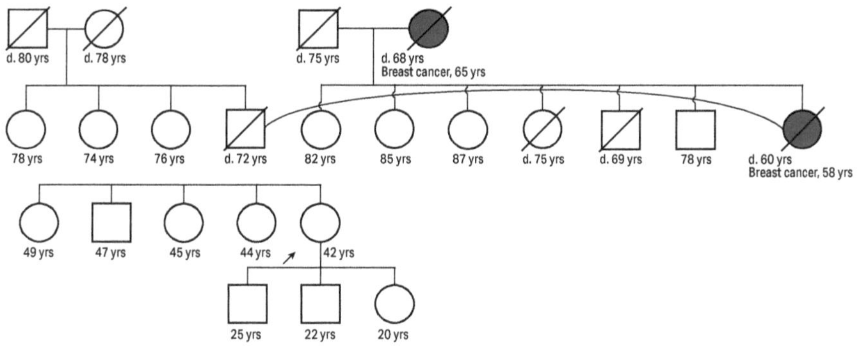

The proband has multiple paternal relatives without a diagnosis of cancer, and the proband's mother has six siblings without a diagnosis of cancer who have lived past middle age. Based on this pedigree, her risk of cancer calculated with the Tyrer-Cuzick model is estimated to be 20%.

Other models calculate the risk of having a pathogenic variant. When the risk is greater than 10%–20%, it is often appropriate to consider genetic testing (Cintolo-Gonzalez et al., 2017; Hampel et al., 2015). Similar to the models that estimate risk of cancer, the models that estimate risk of a pathogenic variant have strengths and limitations. In some cases, these calculations are also required for insurance coverage eligibility (see Figure 3-2).

Some individuals and families are more comfortable with numerical discussions than others. The concept that is most important for individuals and families to understand is how their risk calculation compares to the risk in the general population. The anchor of understanding risk in the general population helps individuals to understand the magnitude of their risk and why recommendations for care may be tailored to their individual situation.

PRETEST COUNSELING

Components of the Genetic Counseling Process

Once the genetics professional evaluates the pedigree and suggests that genetic testing is an option, a thorough discussion of the benefits, risks, and limitations of genetic testing must take place. This discussion is a vital part of the genetic counseling and testing process (Grady et al., 2019).

Cancer genetic counseling must be tailored to the individual psychosocial needs and learning capabilities of each patient. This includes exploration of the motivation for testing, mental health history, socioeconomic considerations, cultural background and beliefs, family dynamics, perceptions, and beliefs about risks.

This usually is a labor-intensive process. Families should anticipate at least one to two sessions lasting 60–90 minutes before testing to ensure that they truly have adequate information to provide informed consent and make a decision that is congruent with their own individual needs. Figure 3-3 outlines activities that typically occur in a cancer genetic counseling session.

Informed Consent

Whether individuals choose to undergo genetic testing or not, they must have enough information to decide what is most appropriate for their personal situations. Because many considerations and consequences are associated with genetic testing, pretest counseling provides the education necessary to making an informed decision that best suits a patient's circumstances.

If an individual opts against testing, the genetics professional will make recommendations for cancer prevention and early detection based on the patient's personal and family medical history. For example, if a patient has a first-degree relative with a history of colon cancer and testing is not performed, the genetics professional may recommend that a colonoscopy be conducted at a younger age and more frequently than typically recommended in the general population.

If someone decides to undergo genetic testing, the genetics professional will have the individual sign a consent form prior to testing. The consent form acknowledges that the patient has had the opportunity to explore the points outlined in Figure 3-4 and has had the opportunity to ask questions. Patients should be given all this information prior to making a testing decision. A patient must consider a great deal of information prior to genetic testing, including the possible outcomes of testing (positive, negative, and noninformative), management strategies, and implications for other family members—noting that the patient is responsible for contacting family members. Informed consent also requires that the patient be educated about risks of developing cancer in the future and risks

FIGURE 3-3 ▪ COMPONENTS OF CANCER GENETIC COUNSELING

- Collection of a detailed family history and pedigree construction
- Collection of information about personal risk factors for developing cancer
- Collection of information about previous cancer screening and results
- Counseling discussion
  - Risks for cancers in the population
  - Individual's risks for a particular cancer based on risk factor assessment
  - Potential genetic pathogenic variants being considered for testing, risk calculations, and clinical criteria linked to those pathogenic variants
  - Factors that limit the interpretation and calculation of risk, such as limited family history, adoption, or incomplete information about family members
  - Identification of the best person to initiate testing in the family
  - Rationale for ordering specific genetic test(s), including technical accuracy, and the rationale for why a specific laboratory was selected
  - Implications of a positive, negative, or noninformative test result: This should include the possibility of having variants of unknown significance. Patients should be informed that, in most cases, these variants are not actionable and do not alter management. Additional testing in other family members is often not possible.
  - Potential prevention and early-detection strategies (risks, benefits, and limitations, depending on the test outcome)
  - Testing alternatives, including no testing
  - Potential risks to other family members and principles of cascade genetic testing
  - Options to enroll in variant or research studies, based on family history
  - Potential discrimination risks for health insurance or employment and federal protection provided by the Genetic Information Nondiscrimination Act (GINA): Discussion should note that GINA does not provide federal protection for life, disability, or long-term care insurance.
  - Strategies to disclose results and information to other at-risk family members
  - Potential psychological risks and benefits of testing
  - Specimen collection: This might include blood, saliva, and occasionally, a skin biopsy for fibroblasts.
  - Fees for testing, counseling, and education
  - Potential costs for testing, including insurance coverage and self-pay options
  - Opportunity to ask questions

of having a pathogenic variant, as well as concepts related to germline genetic transmission. Educating patients prior to testing ensures that when the results become available, the patient will be prepared to deal with the consequences.

Risks and Benefits

Genetic testing offers potential benefits whether the results are positive or negative for a pathogenic variant. Test results can provide a sense of relief from feelings of uncertainty and enable an individual to take positive action in managing health risks. For example, in a family with a known pathogenic variant, a negative result can eliminate the need for multiple frequent screening tests and,

FIGURE 3-4 ▪ COMPONENTS OF INFORMED CONSENT FOR GENETIC TESTING

- Basic concepts of genetic transmission
- Purpose of the genetic test, accuracy of the test, type of specimen required, and testing condition(s)
- Rationale for offering the test, chance of detecting a pathogenic variant, and ideal person in the family to initiate testing
- Potential benefits, risks, and limitations of testing
- Explanation of what test results mean, including positive and negative results, and the potential for uninformative results, including a variant of unknown significance
- Screening options, based on test results
- Available treatment options, depending on test results
- Available counseling and support services for the entire family
- Possible physical or emotional risks associated with the test
- How results might provide information about other family members' health, including the risk of developing a particular condition or the possibility of having affected children
- Availability of coordination of care for other potentially at-risk family members (cascade genetic testing)
- Disclosure of results plan (how, when, to whom)
- Test specimen storage after testing
- Potential research studies available
- Acknowledgment of opportunity provided to discuss the testing process with a knowledgeable genetics professional
- Acknowledgment that the patient was informed of the right to decline testing

in some cases, risk-reducing surgery. A positive result can guide decisions about more intensive cancer prevention, including the possibility of risk-reducing surgery, and cancer screening options.

Many of the risks associated with genetic testing involve the emotional, social, and financial consequences of the test results. Patients may experience anger, depression, anxiety, frustration, fear, or guilt about their results. Depending on the outcome of the results, stress and tension can develop in family dynamics. Learning about adoption or misattributed paternity are genuine risks.

Many patients have concerns about genetic discrimination. The Genetic Information Nondiscrimination Act (GINA) of 2008 is a federal law that protects most Americans from discrimination by health insurance companies and employers with more than 15 employees. However, it does not apply to military health plans, the Veterans Health Administration, or the Indian Health Service. This law prohibits health insurers from using genetic information when deciding who to cover and how much to charge for insurance. GINA prohibits employers from discriminating on the basis of genetic information in hiring, firing or layoffs, pay, or other personnel actions, such as promotions, classifications, or assignments. The law applies no matter how the employers obtain the information (GINA, 2008). The protections of GINA extend to testing results ordered by a professional, as well as those obtained by direct-to-consumer testing (Areheart & Roberts, 2019). GINA does not restrict use of genetic information for life insurance, disability insurance, or long-term care insurance. If individuals want increased coverage for life, disability, or long-term care insurance, they should obtain this insurance before undergoing genetic testing (Underhill-Blazey & Klehm, 2020).

Limitations and Uncertainties

A genetic testing result may provide only limited information about an inherited condition. Many patients are surprised to learn that, even after testing, many unknowns still surround results. For example, a test cannot necessarily determine if a person will show symptoms of a disorder or malignancy, how severe the symptoms will be, or whether the disorder will progress over time. These uncertainties are related to **penetrance**—the proportion of people with a particular pathogenic variant who develop cancer—and **variable expressivity**—the variety of cancers and severity of symptoms that can occur in different family members with the same pathogenic variant. Even if the risk for developing malignancies is high, testing does not provide information about when cancer could develop nor the exact organ site that could be affected.

Another major limitation is the lack of screening, prevention, or treatment strategies for various malignancies associated with a specific altered gene, especially in the less common variants. A genetics professional can explain in detail the benefits, risks, and limitations of a particular test or panel of genes. As stated previously, a patient must understand and consider this possibility among others before proceeding. Patients and families need to clearly understand that, unless a pathogenic variant is identified in a family, the possibility of hereditary predisposition cannot be eliminated. Pretest counseling should include information about the possibility of a variant of unknown significance and that such a result is noninformative and not actionable.

Costs

Because testing can be expensive and insurance reimbursement is variable, providers will often seek prior authorization so that individuals understand their potential financial responsibilities (Whitworth et al., 2017). The cost of genetic testing can range from approximately $150 for a single-site test to more than $6,000 for a panel with many genes (Foote et al., 2017). Many insurance providers, including Medicare and Medicaid, have specific criteria and prior authorization requirements for genetic testing as a covered benefit. Concerns about the costs of genetic testing are very real, and the genetics professional can work with the laboratory and insurance company to try to make genetic testing and counseling affordable.

Genetic Testing Specimens

Genetic testing generally uses a specimen of blood or saliva depending on the test or panel of tests ordered. Patients who have a history of hematologic malignancy may need a skin biopsy to be cultured for fibroblasts to extract DNA (Drazer et al., 2016). Results typically take two to four weeks to be returned, sometimes longer. At the time of specimen collection, the genetics professional will discuss approximately when results will be available and how results will be disclosed.

SELECTION OF HOW AND WHO TO TEST

Selection of the Genetic Test

Although costs are decreasing, genetic testing can be expensive. Selection of the most appropriate test and the best person within the family to test is important to maximize the possibility of obtaining informative test results, to facilitate the most accurate interpretation of results, and to guide testing recommendations for the rest of the family. Many considerations go into the selection. Research clearly demonstrates that involving a genetics professional decreases errors in the interpretation and ordering of genetic testing and also maximizes cost savings (Farmer et al., 2019; Mahon, 2017, 2019).

The genetics professional will carefully examine personal and family history risk factors, consider possible genetic diagnoses, and may suggest genetic testing. This assessment occurs in several different ways. If a model that predicts risk of a germline pathogenic variant estimates a person's risk to be greater than 10%, then it is appropriate to consider genetic testing (LaDuca et al., 2020). NCCN and other organizations also have criteria for when to consider genetic testing (Manahan et al., 2019; NCCN, 2020b).

In the past, genetic testing has typically been focused on one or two genes. However, recent advances in genetics have identified many genes associated with hereditary risk. In most cases, genetic testing in a family now usually includes testing for multiple genes, known as **panel testing**, typically performed with next-generation sequencing (Morganti et al., 2019). A panel may evaluate multiple genes associated with a particular cancer, such as breast or colon cancer. Most genetics professionals will also consider if the panel of genes contains genes that are considered actionable. For a gene to be considered actionable, specific evidence-based recommendations must be available for prevention and early detection of cancer associated with the gene, and when implemented, recommendations are expected to improve an outcome associated with decreased morbidity and mortality.

In the following case, a 23-year-old woman with follicular thyroid cancer was referred for testing. Unfortunately, she has no knowledge of her paternal family history. The maternal side of the family has a significant history of ovarian cancer, early-onset breast cancer, and colorectal cancer.

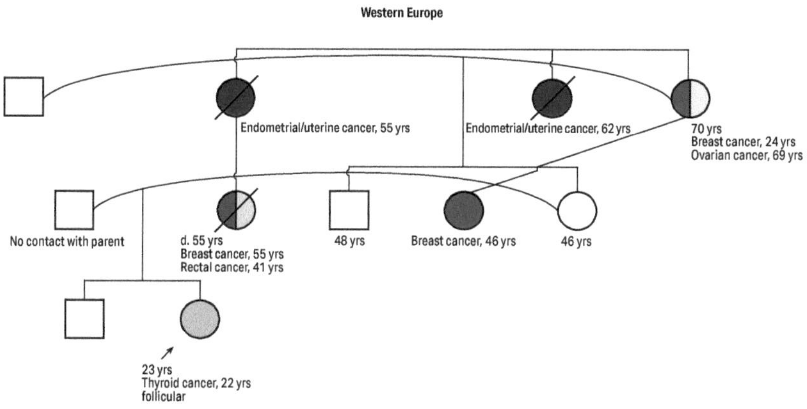

This history could be suggestive of hereditary breast and ovarian cancer syndromes or other conditions, such as Lynch syndrome. Panel testing was selected that included genes associated with both of these syndromes, as well as thyroid cancer syndromes because of the young age at onset. A *CHEK2* pathogenic variant was detected, and it was later detected in her maternal grandmother as well. By focusing on a variety of genes instead of a single syndrome the genetic testing was able to identify a pathogenic variant that is actionable and provides the opportunity for cascade genetic testing in other family members.

If the individual has had genetic testing in the past for one or two genes that did not identify a pathogenic variant, the genetics professional may suggest more expanded testing with a panel to identify a pathogenic variant (King & Mahon, 2017).

Selection of the Best Family Member to Test

If a pathogenic variant has never been identified in the family, the genetics professional will try to identify the best person to initiate testing in the family. Ideally, a family member who has been diagnosed with cancer (known as an *affected person*)—whether in active treatment or living after definitive treatment—has the highest likelihood for a positive result, which will provide helpful information for that person's care, as well as make it possible to test other family members who do not have a diagnosis of cancer. A family member with early-onset disease, bilateral cancers, or a history of multiple cancers is usually the best person to test (see Figure 2-5 for key indicators of hereditary risk). If an affected family member is not available for testing, testing of an unaffected family member can be performed; however, a negative test result will not be as informative and does not necessarily mean that risk is not increased. This potential limitation needs to be carefully discussed prior to testing a nonaffected individual.

In this case, a 49-year-old woman was referred for testing because of a family history of breast cancer. Her mother, who was not open to testing, appeared to be the best person for testing.

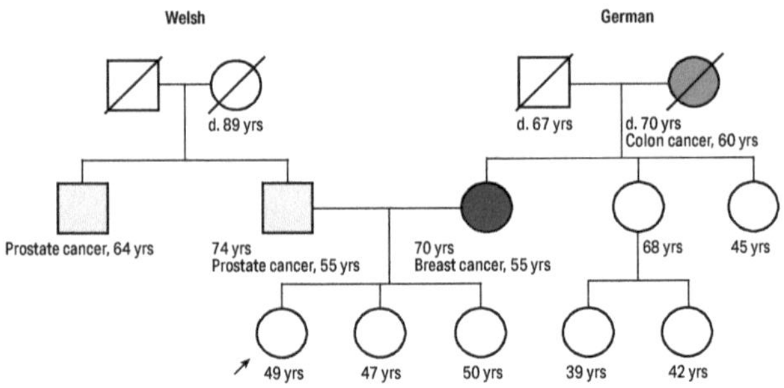

The patient was informed of the possible limitations of testing a nonaffected person. Her risk calculations suggested a breast cancer risk of approximately 22%. The patient had more intensive breast screening, including breast MRI, and was found to have an abnormality that was proven to be an early ductal carcinoma in situ. Given this diagnosis, the patient was now affected and appropriate to test. She was offered genetic testing for *BRCA1* and *BRCA2*, which was clinically available at that time. Testing was negative. The patient continued to follow up to find out if more testing was available. Approximately four years later, she underwent newer panel testing, and a pathogenic *ATM* variant was detected, which likely explains the early-onset breast cancer in the patient, as well as the maternal family history of breast and colon cancer. Selecting the correct individual to test in this family and implementing follow-up testing when it became available enabled the detection of an actionable pathogenic variant and the possibility of informative testing for other family members. This case also illustrates the value of risk assessment to guide screening recommendations. Without the more intensive breast cancer screening with breast MRI, this patient's breast cancer might not have been detected at an early stage.

Once a pathogenic variant is identified in a family, other family members can usually have testing only for the specific identified pathogenic variant. This is referred to as **cascade genetic testing** (Caswell-Jin et al., 2019). In cascade genetic testing, genetic testing for an identified familial pathogenic variant extends to disease-free relatives to enable the implementation of more intensive cancer prevention and early measures in those most likely to benefit and spare those at average risk the expense and potential risks associated with such measures.

The following case illustrates inappropriate use of cascade genetic testing. A 36-year-old woman was referred for explanation of her testing results, which were positive for a pathogenic variant in *BRCA2*. The family has an extensive history of breast cancer and a known *BRCA2* pathogenic variant on the maternal side. The paternal side has only one case of later-onset prostate cancer.

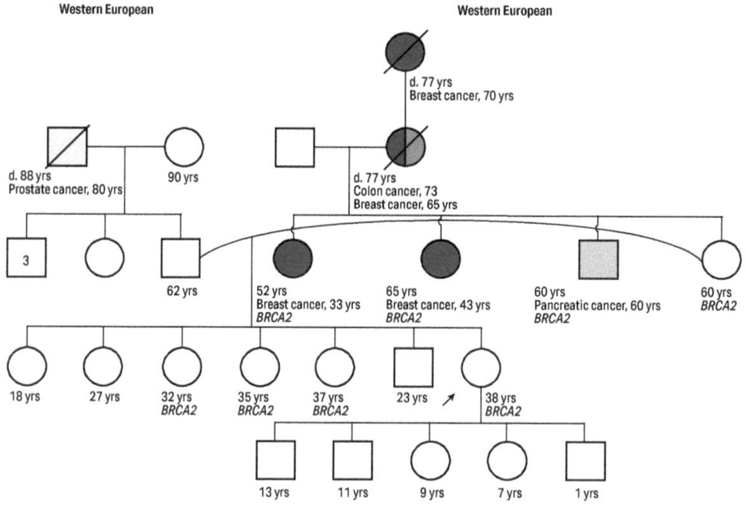

Single-site *BRCA2* testing would have been appropriate for this patient, but her provider ordered a panel of 46 genes for which the patient had a high insurance co-pay. Much less costly single-site testing would have been more than adequate in this situation.

In some cases, more extensive testing is appropriate. In this case, a 37-year-old woman has a known *BRCA2* pathogenic variant on the maternal side. The paternal side has a history of colon, uterine, and pancreatic cancer, which is suggestive of Lynch syndrome or another hereditary colon cancer syndrome.

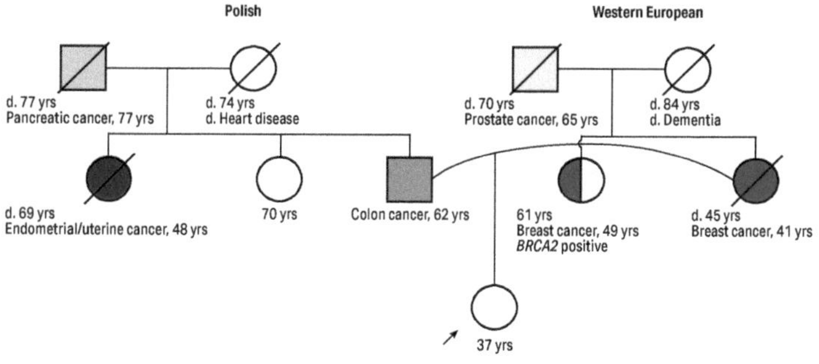

Testing for only the known *BRCA2* pathogenic variant could miss risk from the paternal side. The patient's father has a diagnosis of colon cancer. It would be appropriate to test him first to understand the risk from that side of the family. If her father had been deceased and no other paternal relatives were alive with a diagnosis of cancer, expanded panel testing might be an appropriate consideration.

The following case also illustrates the importance of considering both sides of the family. A 63-year-old woman who was diagnosed with breast cancer at 46 years of age was referred to a genetics provider after her oncologist submitted an order for *BRCA1* and *BRCA2* testing, which was denied. After constructing a three-generation pedigree that included maternal and paternal relatives, it became apparent that three relatives had breast cancer, and three paternal relatives had histories of paragangliomas and pheochromocytomas.

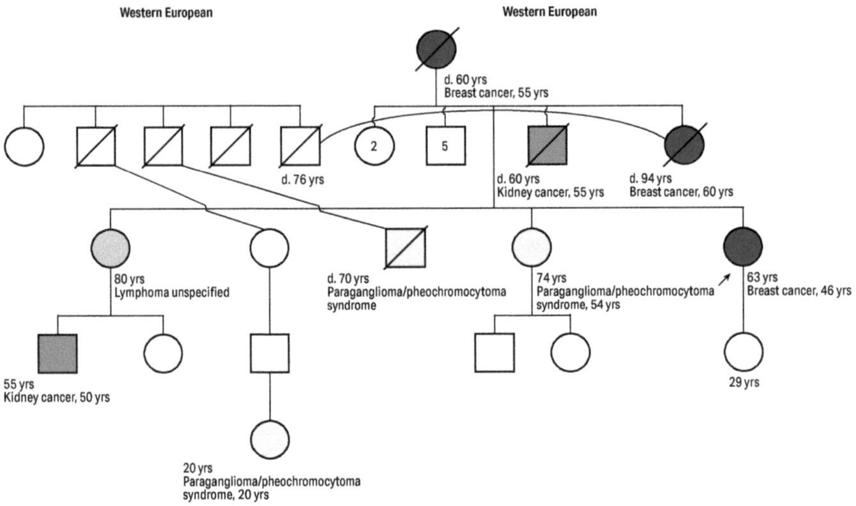

A custom panel of 44 genes was ordered, and the patient was found to have an *SDHD* pathogenic variant associated with paraganglioma/pheochromocytoma syndrome. The patient had extensive screening and was found to have a paraganglioma, which was removed, and testing was offered to other family members. Maternal relatives were instructed to consider more intensive breast cancer screening given the family history of breast cancer, and the family was informed that no pathogenic variants associated with breast cancer were detected.

Every family is unique, and the genetics professional will help the family select the best tests based on the family history. The science of genetics is rapidly changing, and families need to stay in contact with the genetics professional so that they receive the most current and comprehensive care available.

POSSIBLE GENOMIC TESTING RESULTS

The results of genetic tests are not always straightforward and clear, which often makes interpreting and explaining them a challenge. As part of counseling and informed consent, genetic counselors need to educate patients and families about the complexities of interpreting results, as well as give them opportunities to ask questions. When interpreting test results, the genetics professional considers a person's medical history, family history, and the type of genetic test.

Once a genetic test has detected a pathogenic variant in a family, it is possible to calculate the statistical risk of other family members having the same pathogenic variant based on the relationship to the person who carries the pathogenic variant. In the case of autosomal dominance, first-degree relatives (children, siblings, and parents) have a 50% chance of having inherited the variant (Gunder McClary, 2020). Second-degree relatives (grandparents, aunts, and uncles) have a 25% chance of having the pathogenic variant. If a pathogenic variant is not detected in the family, calculating the risks of developing cancers can be helpful in recommending a plan for prevention and early detection.

For the first person tested in a family, a spectrum of results is possible. Laboratories do not typically report common or benign changes. They report variants classified as likely benign, of unknown significance, likely pathogenic, or pathogenic (see Figure 3-5). Reported pathogenic and likely pathogenic variants, if actionable, can provide valuable information related to cancer prevention and early-detection recommendations. In the case of a variant of unknown significance, it is not clear what kind of risk the variant imposes.

Positive Result

A **positive result** indicates that the test identified a pathogenic variant or a **likely pathogenic variant** that increases the risk for developing cancer. Knowledge of this increased cancer risk can assist in making medical management and treatment decisions with the goals of early detection and cancer prevention. In the case of a positive result, healthcare providers may make certain recommendations, such as the following:

- Start screening earlier than usually recommended.
- Screen more often than usually recommended.

FIGURE 3-5 ▪ POSSIBLE CLASSIFICATIONS IN GENETIC TESTING RESULTS

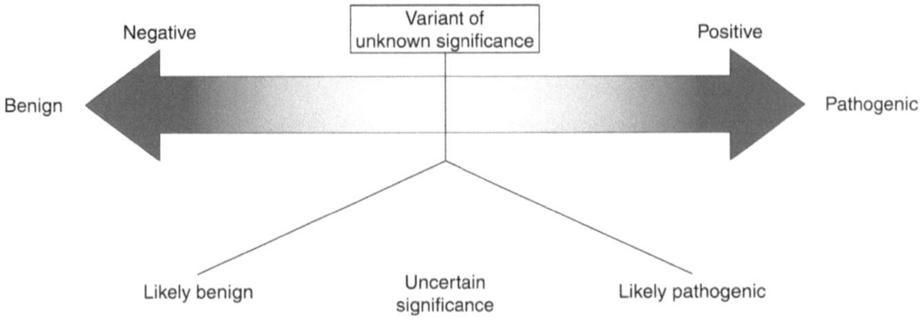

This illustration demonstrates the range of possible classifications of a genetic testing result in which some variants are clearly positive (harmful) and some are negative (clearly harmless). However, the variant of unknown significance might be unclear if it is harmful or harmless or leaning toward benign and pathogenic.

- Screen with tests that are used only for people known to be at increased risk.
- Monitor closely for signs or symptoms of cancer and promptly evaluate any change.
- Learn about options to help reduce the risk of certain cancers, which may include medications or preventive surgery.
- Adopt a healthier lifestyle, including smoking cessation, healthier diet, exercise, limitation of alcohol consumption, and reduction of exposure to ultraviolet light.

Negative Results

Two types of negative results are possible. A **noninformative negative result** occurs when the first person tested in a family does not have a pathogenic variant. This is clearly a limitation of testing that must be discussed in pre- and post-test counseling. Although the person tested negative for known pathogenic variants in whatever genes were tested, this result does not necessarily mean that there is no hereditary risk. It could mean that the family does not have a hereditary risk, or it could mean that the family has another pathogenic variant for which testing was not ordered or is not yet available. Recommendations for care for the individual and other family members will be based on personal and family medical histories and risk factors.

For families with a known pathogenic variant, a **true negative result** indicates that the individual tested has not inherited the pathogenic variant. A true negative result does not mean a person has no risk of developing cancer. Instead, the person has at least an average risk for developing cancer and can follow standard population-based recommendations for the prevention and early detection of cancer (American Cancer Society, 2020). A true negative result can help ease uncertainty and provide a sense of relief.

Variant of Unknown Significance

A **variant of unknown significance** indicates that the test detected a change in the genetic material, but it is not clear if the change material is harmless or harmful. Sometimes, information about a genetic change is limited, especially in "newer," more recently discovered genes, and it cannot yet be classified as harmful or harmless. Because the meaning of the variant is unclear, recommendations for care should be based on the individual and family medical histories and risk factors (Morganti et al., 2019).

To further clarify the clinical meaning of a variant, sometimes testing family members who have or had cancer may be helpful, but only in the context of a variant reclassification study, usually offered by the testing laboratory. Participation in such studies does not usually result in a quick reclassification of a variant and typically takes years before the variant is seen in enough families to understand its meaning. Reputable testing laboratories have large teams of scientists who are constantly reviewing data on variants of unknown significance, but it can be a slow process. If the variant continues to be found in family members with related cancers, in addition to other evidence, the variant may be reclassified as a pathogenic variant. At that time, genetic testing for the pathogenic variant can then be offered to other family members. In other situations, the variant is reclassified as harmless. Until a variant is reclassified, recommendations for cancer prevention and early detection are based on personal medical history and family history.

Patients are often confused and frustrated when their test report states that one or more gene variants of unknown significance were detected (Colas et al., 2019). With the current panels, the probability of detecting a variant of unknown significance is significantly higher than the probability of detecting a harmful pathogenic variant, and patients and families need to be prepared for this possibility. Research suggests that 80%–90% of variants of unknown significance are ultimately reclassified as likely benign (Mersch et al., 2018). When the test report shows one or more variants of unknown significance, patients and families often need more education about the meaning of the result and the rationale for care recommendations. Most genetics professionals will recommend that the patient follow up annually to learn if more is known about the variant, to review the personal and family medical histories for changes, and to determine if recommendations for care are still current.

In the following case, a family has multiple instances of early-onset breast cancer and colon cancer. In addition, no information about the paternal side of the family is available. A panel of genes was ordered, and a pathogenic variant of *BRCA1* was detected, as well as three variants of unknown significance in the *APC*, *MSH6*, and *SMAD4* genes.

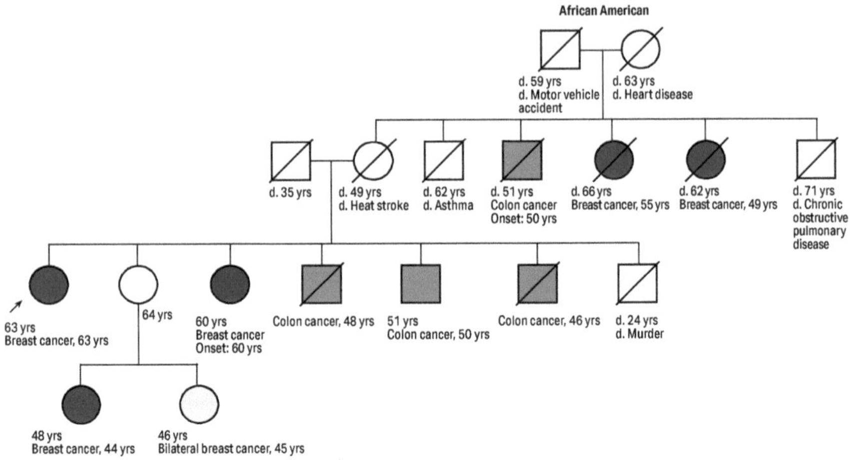

Other family members could have testing for the known *BRCA1* pathogenic variant, and those who test positive would receive recommendations for more intensive screening and risk-reducing mastectomies and oophorectomies. All family members, regardless of the testing results for the *BRCA1* pathogenic variant, were advised to have a colonoscopy every three years, or more frequently if polyps were detected, because of the extensive history of colon cancer. Some family members were offered the option of participating in a variant reclassification study. Testing was not recommended for the variants of unknown significance as the meaning of the variants is not clear.

AFTER GENOMIC TESTING

Ideally, after genetic testing has been completed, a genetics professional provides the results during an in-person appointment, but sometimes patients choose to receive results by phone or through videoconferencing. Telephone disclosure of test results has been increasingly used to reduce time and travel burdens on patients and to improve access to care (Mahon, 2020). The plan for disclosure should be discussed at the time the specimen is sent. Along with a copy of the results, the genetics professional also usually writes a letter that summarizes what the findings mean for the patient, what other family members should do, and specific recommendations for cancer prevention and early detection. The patient can share these materials with other healthcare providers.

The genetics professional will also help coordinate care for the rest of the family and can assist with finding a genetics professional located near other family members. In addition, the genetics professional can offer guidance to individuals on how best to reach out to other family members and reinforce why it is so essential (Mahon, 2019). Genetic testing requires long-term follow-up to ensure the best care possible for the individual and family and to ensure that recommendations for care remain current.

Nurses must also play a role after genetic testing by informing patients that recommendations for prevention and early detection may change. Care plans could change if a genetic variant is reclassified as a pathogenic variant and if research reveals more about different genetic variants. Also, newer methods of cancer prevention and early detection may become available. Genetics professionals can help individuals understand options and coordinate care with other healthcare providers. Genetics professionals are also a great source of information on new research. More testing could become available, allowing for families with no previously detected pathogenic variant to learn more about their genetic risks. Because the field of genetics changes rapidly, people who have undergone genetic testing or counseling should follow up annually with their genetics professional, at least by phone, for any changes in care recommendations. For example, in the early 2000s women with a known *BRCA2* pathogenic variant were advised to consider risk-reducing mastectomies and oophorectomies after their childbearing years were complete because the known risks at that time associated with *BRCA2* were elevated breast and ovarian cancer. More recently, *BRCA2* pathogenic variants have also been found to be associated with increased risk for developing pancreatic, prostate, and possibly melanoma cancers (NCCN, 2020a). For this reason, people with these pathogenic variants should check every 12–18 months to determine if their recommendations for care are still appropriate.

Adjustment to a diagnosis of hereditary cancer syndrome can take time, and patients and families can have many different reactions, including anger, anxiety, and depression (Yanes et al., 2019). Some patients find that joining a support group can be helpful. Those families and individuals who have difficulty adjusting to the diagnosis of hereditary cancer syndrome may benefit from counseling.

IMPLICATIONS FOR FAMILY MEMBERS

In the event that a pathogenic variant has not been detected in the family or a variant of unknown significance has been discovered, other family members may still be at increased risk for developing cancer. In this case, the genetics professional will make recommendations for other family members based on their medical history and the family medical history of cancer.

Many emotions and unexpected consequences can surface when families learn the results of genetic testing. Learning that an individual or individuals in a family are at increased risk for developing cancer can be frightening and upsetting. Parents sometimes feel guilty or worry about passing on the pathogenic variant to their children. Other times, people can feel relief, even in the face of a positive test result. A positive test allows individuals to begin selecting a plan for cancer prevention and early detection that is more likely to be effective.

News of a negative test can have the same affect. Family members may find comfort in learning that they did not inherit the risk or that their offspring cannot inherit the pathogenic variant. However, those feelings of relief may turn to guilt if other family members test positive, while they, themselves, have an average risk. In some cases, family members do not want to know if they are at increased risk, especially if they can do little about it or do not want to undergo more drastic preventive measures, such as surgery. Family members should know they have the option to test, but each family member must decide individually. A genetics professional can help the patient and family cope with this wide range of emotions, including handling those who do not wish to be tested.

If a pathogenic variant is detected, the healthcare provider cannot directly contact relatives and inform them of the possibility of having increased risk. This limitation is discussed during pretest counseling, so patients understand those who undergo testing are responsible for contacting other family members to inform them of potential risk and to encourage them to contact a genetics professional (Caswell-Jin et al., 2019). Genetics professionals can assist with this process by identifying which relatives should be informed. Relaying this kind of sensitive information can be difficult, especially if family relationships are strained. Genetics professionals can teach patients about strategies to disclose this information to other family members. Sometimes testing reveals family secrets, such as paternity, adoptions, or other uncomfortable issues. Before starting the process of testing, families need to be made aware that genetic testing can come with complications.

Clearly, genetic testing can be complex for many members of a family. Genetics professionals can assist family members in working through these issues and help each family member make the most appropriate decision. For these reasons, people who are considering genetic testing should speak with a genetics professional about these issues prior to testing (King & Mahon, 2017). See Table 3-1.

SUMMARY

Understanding issues related to hereditary cancer syndromes is an important component of nursing practice. Providing care to patients and families with suspected or known germline genetic risk for developing cancer involves an interprofessional team. Involvement of a credentialed genetics professional in this care decreases errors in the interpretation and ordering of genetic testing and also maximizes cost savings (Farmer et al., 2019). All nurses, regardless of practice setting and roles, have a responsibility to refer patients to a genetics profes-

TABLE 3-1 ▪ POTENTIAL OUTCOMES OF GENETIC TESTING

Result	Implications for Individuals	Implications for Family	Other Implications
Positive result	Individuals have increased risk of developing cancer. Patients should adopt a healthier lifestyle, including stopping smoking, eating healthier, exercising, limiting alcohol consumption, and reducing exposure to ultraviolet light. Patients can consider having risk-reducing surgery or using chemoprevention agents. Positive result enables individuals to make decisions about prevention and early detection.	First-degree relatives have a 50% chance of having the pathogenic variant. Single-site testing would clarify if the family member has the pathogenic variant and associated increased risk. Single-site testing has a lower cost.	Positive result does not inform about what type of cancer will develop or when, only that the risk is higher. Relevant cancer screening should start earlier than usually recommended. Relevant cancer screening should occur more often than that usually recommended. Patients can be screened with tests that are recommended only for people known to be at increased risk. Providers should monitor closely for signs or symptoms of cancer and promptly evaluate any change.
True negative (no pathogenic variant detected in an individual of a family with a known pathogenic variant)	In most cases, these people will not need screening greater than that recommended for the general population and should receive information about the importance of a healthy lifestyle to prevent cancer. Individuals do not need to consider risk-reducing surgery or chemoprevention.	Offspring from this individual are not at risk for carrying the known pathogenic variant. No further testing is necessary. Unless offspring have risk from the other parent, their risk for developing cancer is probably similar to that of the general population. Following guidelines for the general population for prevention and early detection is appropriate.	True negative provides a more accurate cancer risk assessment. True negative provides psychological relief regarding risk for developing cancer and that offspring will not inherit the pathogenic variant.

(Continued on next page)

TABLE 3-1 ▪ POTENTIAL OUTCOMES OF GENETIC TESTING *(CONTINUED)*

Result	Implications for Individuals	Implications for Family	Other Implications
Negative result (no pathogenic variant identified in family)	Negative results usually occur when the first individual in a family is tested. The cancer may be the result of a different pathogenic variant from the one tested, or the cancer seen in the family occurs because of nonhereditary reasons. Results are difficult to interpret and must be considered in conjunction with personal risk factors and family history.	Testing is not typically available to other unaffected members in the family because they will also likely test negative. The cancer may be the result of a different pathogenic variant from the one tested, or the cancer seen in the family occurs because of nonhereditary reasons.	The best options for cancer prevention and early detection are not always clear. Individuals may consider participating in research studies or high-risk registries.
Genetic variant of unknown significance	Test identifies a change in the genetic material; it is not clear if it is a harmless or harmful change. Results do not provide meaningful information. The test result is not actionable.	Meaningful testing will not be available to other family members.	Results may create uncertainty and anxiety about the usefulness of cancer-risk reduction strategies. Results require formulation of recommendations for cancer prevention and detection based on personal risk factors and family history, with careful consideration of potential benefits and risks. Individuals may consider participation in a research study or hereditary cancer registry.

Note. Based on information from Colas et al., 2019; Grady et al., 2019; King & Mahon, 2017; LaDuca et al., 2020.

sional, support patients and families, and understand the influence of genetics and genomics in health care. All nurses need to be able to elicit a family history, identify patients who might benefit from testing, and educate patients on how testing can be helpful in decision-making. Once a patient receives counseling from a genetics professional, nurses need to ascertain that the patient understands recommendations for care and offer to assist with carrying out the recommendations. Care based on genomic information is constantly changing, and nurses need to work with genetics professionals to be certain that recommendations are still correct and appropriate. After undergoing genetic testing or consultation with a genetics professional, individuals can turn to and often will seek out nurses who can provide education, support, coordination of care, and assistance with the prevention and risk reduction plan.

REFERENCES

American Cancer Society. (2019). *Cancer prevention and early detection facts and figures 2019–2020.* https://www.cancer.org/research/cancer-facts-statistics/cancer-prevention-early-detection.html

American Cancer Society. (2020). *Cancer facts and figures 2020.* https://www.cancer.org/research/cancer-facts-statistics/all-cancer-facts-figures/cancer-facts-figures-2020.html

Areheart, B.A., & Roberts, J.L. (2019). GINA, big data, and the future of employee privacy. *Yale Law Journal, 128*(3), 710–790

Boehm, L., Weisberg, T., Linendoll, N., Damon, A.C., Erban, J.K., & Parsons, S.K. (2019). Development of phase-specific breast cancer survivorship care plans. *Clinical Breast Cancer, 19*(6), e723–e730. https://doi.org/10.1016/j.clbc.2019.05.017

Caswell-Jin, J.L., Zimmer, A.D., Stedden, W., Kingham, K.E., Zhou, A.Y., & Kurian, A.W. (2019). Cascade genetic testing of relatives for hereditary cancer risk: Results of an online initiative. *Journal of the National Cancer Institute, 111*(1), 95–98. https://doi.org/10.1093/jnci/djy147

Cintolo-Gonzalez, J.A., Braun, D., Blackford, A.L., Mazzola, E., Acar, A., Plichta, J.K., ... Hughes, K.S. (2017). Breast cancer risk models: A comprehensive overview of existing models, validation, and clinical applications. *Breast Cancer Research and Treatment, 164*(2), 263–284. https://doi.org/10.1007/s10549-017-4247-z

Cleophat, J.E., Nabi, H., Pelletier, S., Bouchard, K., & Dorval, M. (2018). What characterizes cancer family history collection tools? A critical literature review. *Current Oncology, 25*(4), e335–e350. https://doi.org/10.3747/co.25.4042

Colas, C., Golmard, L., de Pauw, A., Caputo, S.M., & Stoppa-Lyonnet, D. (2019). "Decoding hereditary breast cancer" benefits and questions from multigene panel testing. *Breast, 45,* 29–35. https://doi.org/10.1016/j.breast.2019.01.002

Drazer, M.W., Feurstein, S., West, A.H., Jones, M.F., Churpek, J.E., & Godley, L.A. (2016). How I diagnose and manage individuals at risk for inherited myeloid malignancies. *Blood, 128*(14), 1800–1813. https://doi.org/10.1182/blood-2016-05-670240

Farmer, M.B., Bonadies, D.C., Mahon, S.M., Baker, M.J., Ghate, S.M., Munro, C., ... Matloff, E.T. (2019). Errors in genetic testing: The fourth case series. *Cancer Journal, 25*(4), 231–236. https://doi.org/10.1097/PPO.0000000000000391

Foote, J.R., Lopez-Acevedo, M., Buchanan, A.H., Secord, A.A., Lee, P.S., Fountain, C., ... Havrilesky, L.J. (2017). Cost comparison of genetic testing strategies in women with epithelial ovarian cancer. *Journal of Oncology Practice, 13*(2), e120–e129. https://doi.org/10.1200/jop.2016.011866

Genetic Information Nondiscrimination Act of 2008, Pub. L. No. 110-233, 122 Stat. 881. (2008).

Grady, M.C., Kolla, K.A., & Peshkin, B.N. (2019). Multigene cancer panels: Implications for pre- and post-test genetic counseling. *Current Genetic Medicine Reports, 7*(4), 169–179. https://doi.org/10.1007/s40142-019-00173-8

Gunder McClary, L.M. (2020). *Essentials of medical genetics for nursing and health professionals: An interprofessional approach.* Jones and Bartlett Learning.

Hampel, H., Bennett, R.L., Buchanan, A., Pearlman, R., & Wiesner, G.L. (2015). A practice guideline from the American College of Medical Genetics and Genomics and the National Society of Genetic Counselors: Referral indications for cancer predisposition assessment. *Genetics in Medicine, 17*(1), 70–87. https://doi.org/10.1038/gim.2014.147

King, E., & Mahon, S.M. (2017). Genetic testing: Challenges and changes in testing for hereditary cancer syndromes. *Clinical Journal of Oncology Nursing, 21*(5), 589–598. https://doi.org/10.1188/17.CJON.589-598

LaDuca, H., Polley, E.C., Yussuf, A., Hoang, L., Gutierrez, S., Hart, S.N., ... Dolinsky, J.S. (2020). A clinical guide to hereditary cancer panel testing: Evaluation of gene-specific cancer associations and sensitivity of genetic testing criteria in a cohort of 165,000 high-risk patients. *Genetics in Medicine, 22*(2), 407–415. https://doi.org/10.1038/s41436-019-0633-8

Lu, K.H., Wood, M.E., Daniels, M., Burke, C., Ford, J., Kauff, N.D., ... Hughes, K.S. (2014). American Society of Clinical Oncology expert statement: Collection and use of a cancer family history for oncology providers. *Journal of Clinical Oncology, 32*(8), 833–840. https://doi.org/10.1200/JCO.2013.50.9257

Mahon, S.M. (2013). Allocation of work activities in a comprehensive cancer genetics program. *Clinical Journal of Oncology Nursing, 17*(4), 397–404. https://doi.org/10.1188/13.CJON.397-404

Mahon, S.M. (2016). The three-generation pedigree: A critical tool in cancer genetics care. *Oncology Nursing Forum, 43*(5), 655–660. https://doi.org/10.1188/16.ONF.655-660

Mahon, S.M. (2017). Errors in genetic testing: Common causes and strategies for prevention. *Clinical Journal of Oncology Nursing, 21*(6), 673–676. https://doi.org/10.1188/17.CJON.673-676

Mahon, S.M. (2019). Coordination of genetic care: More important and complicated than it seems. *Journal of the National Comprehensive Cancer Network, 17*(11), 1272–1276. https://doi.org/10.6004/jnccn.2019.7343

Mahon, S.M. (2020). Considerations for the telephone disclosure of genetic test results to patients with cancer. *Clinical Journal of Oncology Nursing, 24*(1), 8. https://doi.org/10.1188/20.CJON.8

Manahan, E.R., Kuerer, H.M., Sebastian, M., Hughes, K.S., Boughey, J.C., Euhus, D.M., ... Taylor, W.A. (2019). Consensus guidelines on genetic testing for hereditary breast cancer from the American Society of Breast Surgeons. *Annals of Surgical Oncology, 26*(10), 3025–3031. https://doi.org/10.1245/s10434-019-07549-8

Mersch, J., Brown, N., Pirzadeh-Miller, S., Mundt, E., Cox, H.C., Brown, K., ... Ross, T. (2018). Prevalence of variant reclassification following hereditary cancer genetic testing. *JAMA, 320*(12), 1266–1274. https://doi.org/10.1001/jama.2018.13152

Morganti, S., Tarantino, P., Ferraro, E., D'Amico, P., Viale, G., Trapani, D., ... Curigliano, G. (2019). Complexity of genome sequencing and reporting: Next generation sequencing (NGS) technologies and implementation of precision medicine in real life. *Critical Reviews in Oncology/Hematology, 133,* 171–182. https://doi.org/10.1016/j.critrevonc.2018.11.008

National Comprehensive Cancer Network. (2020a). *NCCN Clinical Practice Guidelines in Oncology (NCCN Guidelines®): Genetic/familial high-risk assessment: Breast, ovarian, and pancreatic* [v.2.2021]. https://www.nccn.org/professionals/physician_gls/pdf/genetics_bop.pdf

National Comprehensive Cancer Network. (2020b). *NCCN Clinical Practice Guidelines in Oncology (NCCN Guidelines®): Genetic/familial high-risk assessment: Colorectal* [v.1.2020]. https://www.nccn.org/professionals/physician_gls/pdf/genetics_colon.pdf

Shane-Carson, K., & Jeter, J.M. (2019). Hereditary risk for cancer. In D.S. Alberts & L.M. Hess (Eds.), *Fundamentals of cancer prevention* (4th ed., pp. 161–197). Springer. https://doi.org/10.1007/978-3-030-15935-1_6

Underhill-Blazey, M., & Klehm, M.R. (2020). Genetic discrimination: The Genetic Information Nondiscrimination Act's impact on practice and research. *Clinical Journal of Oncology Nursing, 24*(2), 135–137. https://doi.org/10.1188/20.CJON.135-137

Whitworth, P., Beitsch, P., Arnell, C., Cox, H.C., Brown, K., Kidd, J., & Lancaster, J.M. (2017). Impact of payer constraints on access to genetic testing. *Journal of Oncology Practice, 13*(1), e47–e56. https://doi.org/10.1200/jop.2016.013581

Yanes, T., Willis, A.M., Meiser, B., Tucker, K.M., & Best, M. (2019). Psychosocial and behavioral outcomes of genomic testing in cancer: A systematic review. *European Journal of Human Genetics, 27*(1), 28–35. https://doi.org/10.1038/s41431-018-0257-5

CHAPTER 4

Direct-to-Consumer Genetic Testing

INTRODUCTION

Genetic testing has moved into the public realm, and individuals can order various types of genetic testing online without an order from or guidance of a healthcare provider. Although direct-to-consumer testing and testing ordered by a healthcare provider are both types of genetic testing, the process for ordering, the types of tests available, and the implications for care are very different (Mahon, 2016).

Unlike tests ordered through a healthcare provider, direct-to-consumer genetic testing (DTCGT) is marketed directly to the general public through multiple venues, including television, print advertisements, and the Internet. The intent of directly interacting with the consumer is to increase accessibility to genetic testing for a wide variety of health conditions, ancestry data, and physical human traits (Gill et al., 2018).

More specific medical genetic testing is typically used to understand a specific health risk or condition and requires an order from a healthcare provider. Ideally, testing follows counseling about the strengths, limitations, and risks of testing, as well as information regarding how test results might inform care. Consumers can also choose a hybrid form of testing. In this scenario, the consumer initiates the process, and after some counseling from a healthcare provider employed by a laboratory, genetic testing is ordered. This is an ever-growing and changing industry. Each form of testing has its own inherent strengths and weaknesses. An understanding of the differences between these types of tests is important so that nurses can provide education and support to patients and families seeking information about these tests. See Table 4-1.

EFFECTS OF DIRECT-TO-CONSUMER GENETIC TESTING

DTCGT generated more than $954 million in revenue in 2019 (AP News, 2020). Regulatory oversight of DTCGT is uneven at best, and at worst, it can

TABLE 4-1 ▪ COMPARISON OF PROVIDER-ORDERED, CONSUMER-INITIATED, AND DIRECT-TO-CONSUMER TESTING OPTIONS

Component	Provider-Initiated Testing	Consumer-Initiated Testing	Direct-to-Consumer Testing
Initiation	Provider recommends, orders, and coordinates testing.	Patient initiates but laboratory provider orders testing.	Consumer selects and orders test. Healthcare provider is not involved.
Testing process	Diagnostic testing includes sequencing of full genes based on the personal and family medical history.	Diagnostic testing includes sequencing of full genes based on standardized panels.	Testing includes specific variants and single nucleotide polymorphisms.
Payment	Testing is typically covered by insurance if diagnostic criteria are satisfied.	Testing may be covered by insurance.	Consumer pays cost when testing is ordered.
Accreditation and regulation	Laboratories will always have CLIA certification and CAP accreditation.	Laboratories may have CLIA certification and CAP accreditation.	Companies may not have CLIA certification and CAP accreditation, and positive results usually must be confirmed in a laboratory with CLIA certification and CAP accreditation. Tests are regulated as a consumer product.
Quality measures	Positive test results are typically confirmed with additional testing in the laboratory with a built-in process.	Positive test results may be confirmed with additional testing in the laboratory.	Companies may not confirm findings.
Support for interpretation of report	Support is available and an expected component of care.	Availability of support depends on the laboratory and testing performed. It is generally available to some extent.	Support is very limited. A customer receives a standardized report with recommendations by email. Some laboratories offer the option of brief counseling with a professional.

(Continued on next page)

TABLE 4-1 ▪ COMPARISON OF PROVIDER-ORDERED, CONSUMER-INITIATED, AND DIRECT-TO-CONSUMER TESTING OPTIONS *(CONTINUED)*

Component	Provider-Initiated Testing	Consumer-Initiated Testing	Direct-to-Consumer Testing
Coordination of care for other family members who may be at risk	Coordination is a standard component of care.	Coordination is usually not available.	Coordination is not available.
Types of testing	Testing is predictive for risk of disease, pharmacogenomics, and carrier testing.	Testing is predictive for risk of disease, pharmacogenomics. and carrier testing.	Testing is limited in predicting for risk of disease, pharmacogenomics, and carrier testing. Testing includes ancestry and other types, such as paternity or curiosity.
Secondary use of data	Data may be used for health research about the genes and variants tested. Additional use of data would require specific consent from the patient to participate in a different study.	Data may be used for health research about the genes and variants tested.	Companies profit from selling of data for secondary analysis.

CAP—College of American Pathologists; CLIA—Clinical Laboratory Improvement Amendments

Note. Based on information from Allyse et al., 2018; Horton et al., 2019; Ramos & Weissman, 2018; Schleit et al., 2019.

be confusing for healthcare providers and consumers. In the United States, the Clinical Laboratory Improvement Amendments (CLIA) of 1988 require that laboratories providing DTCGT results are to be certified and are to employ certain basic practices. However, despite the regulation, there is no assurance that DTCGT results will offer clinical validity or utility. Oversight by the U.S. Food and Drug Administration (FDA) applies to regulation of testing for genetic diseases with testing kits, which are marketed and sold to laboratories for use in medical testing procedures. The Federal Trade Commission is responsible for ensuring that DTCGT advertising is honest and not misleading.

The process and availability of DTCGTs has evolved over more than a decade. Until 2006, only healthcare professionals could order genetic testing. This all changed in 2006 when 23andMe® was launched as the first DTCGT (Stoeklé et al., 2016). As of 2018, more than 10 million people have had genotyping completed (Khan & Mittelman, 2018).

Despite its popularity, however, in 2013, FDA ordered 23andMe to stop offering genetic screening that claimed to assess genetic health risks (Wynn & Chung, 2017). As the basis for the order, FDA cited the lack of clinical validity and concerns that false-positive or false-negative results could lead to unnecessary or delayed care. In April 2017, in a partial reversal of the 2013 order, FDA authorized 23andMe's inclusion of the three Ashkenazi Jewish *BRCA1* and *BRCA2* founder pathogenic variants in its test panel, following a request and documentation from 23andMe that these variants were well established as significant risk factors for developing breast, ovarian, and other cancers (Wynn & Chung, 2017). This FDA approval has raised concerns about the clinical standards to which DTCGT will be held in the future. The FDA ruling exempts other 23andMe genetic health risk tests from premarket review, and companies offering similar tests may be able to forgo regulatory review after submitting the first premarket notification. These actions marked a major shift in FDA policy and opens the door for broad use of DTCGT.

HOW IS DIRECT-TO-CONSUMER GENETIC TESTING ACCOMPLISHED?

DTCGT can be completed without leaving the home or engaging with a healthcare provider. DTCGT kits are easily purchased online, and customers can choose from a variety of products. After the purchase, the customer receives a test kit from the testing company with instructions for collecting a saliva sample. The customer then returns the saliva sample. The saliva sample contains buccal cells, from which DNA is extracted. When results are available, the customer can download them directly from a secure website. Proponents of DTCGT emphasize that this process allows the public easy access to their genetic information without necessarily involving a healthcare provider or health insurance company in the process (Mahon, 2018).

DTCGT is an expanding business, and tests for multiple purposes are available (see Figure 4-1). Commonly utilized tests frequently identify single-nucleotide polymorphisms (SNPs) to make predictions about health, provide information about common traits, and provide information about a person's ancestry. Some DTCGT is very specific, such as paternity tests, but other services provide a broad range of information. DTCGT may combine many different common variants across the genome to place someone in a broad risk category. For example, a report could state that certain genes predispose a person to weigh 6% more than average. This is a **polygenic risk score** (Horton et al., 2019). In DTCGT, the validity, predictability, and clinical utility of these risk scores is often unknown. The scores may be relevant for a very broad health condition, such as heart disease or obesity. In clinical genetic testing, healthcare professionals can employ polygenetic risk scores to estimate the chance of a very specific event, such as risk of breast cancer recur-

FIGURE 4-1 ▪ TYPES OF DIRECT-TO-CONSUMER GENETIC TESTING

- **Health conditions:** Results provide an estimate of the probability of developing common diseases or carrier status for diseases such as cystic fibrosis, Alzheimer disease, and rare genetic conditions. Results can also explain genetic variations related to health-related traits, such as eye color or metabolism. Some companies offer testing for some single specific pathogenic variants associated with developing breast cancer, such as the three common *BRCA1* and *BRCA2* founder pathogenic variants that exist in people of Ashkenazi Jewish ancestry, but not full sequencing of the genes. Some companies offer testing to identify genetic variants that affect drug metabolism. Others offer carrier status testing.
- **Ancestry:** The results of ancestry tests provide clues about where a person's ancestors may have come from, their ethnicity, and genetic connections between families. This testing looks for common genetic variations among people. The greater the number of genetic variations two people have in common, the more likely they are closely related. This type of testing usually involves examining Y chromosome variations, mitochondrial DNA, and single nucleotide polymorphisms (SNPs). For males, it is possible to look for variations in the Y chromosome, which is passed exclusively from father to son, to explore ancestry in the male line. Males and females have mitochondrial DNA, which is passed from the mother, so examining the mitochondrial DNA can be helpful in evaluating maternal ancestry. SNPs are also utilized by comparing SNPs commonly associated with various ethnic groups. Ancestry testing is made by comparing the customer's results with other results in a database. Depending on the size and diversity of the database, results can be quite variable. Many companies that offer this type of testing provide online forums and other services to allow people who have been tested to share and discuss their results with others, which may allow them to discover previously unknown relationships.
- **Kinship:** The results of kinship tests can indicate whether tested individuals are biologically related to one another (e.g., paternity testing).
- **Lifestyle:** The results of lifestyle genetic tests are touted to provide information about lifestyle factors, including food preferences, sleep habits, skin types, and fitness, based on the presence or absence of SNPs. Some of the companies that offer this kind of testing also sell services, products, or programs that can be customized for the individual customer based on test results.

rence with or without the addition of chemotherapy. Risk scores developed by healthcare professionals are based on extensive research and normative data and are recommended as a standard of care by professional organizations.

BENEFITS, RISKS, AND LIMITATIONS OF DIRECT-TO-CONSUMER GENETIC TESTING

Benefits

Despite the limitations of DTCGT and misgivings by some healthcare professionals, there are known benefits to DTCGT. First, the extensive marketing of these tests has raised general public awareness of genetic diseases. Such marketing campaigns have the potential to make consumers aware of potential health risks so that they can take proactive steps to reduce risk. DTCGT is also a more efficient process and provides customers the convenience of ordering a test at any time, without a medical prescription. In addition, companies that provide DTCGT offer an easy and convenient system for delivering results. Consumers are not forced to deal with long wait times for appointments with healthcare providers to have tests ordered for them. In some instances, especially with the hybrid models in which the consumer initiates testing, DTCGT offers access to a professional who can explain the meaning of the results.

Risks and Limitations

One of the biggest risks of DTCGT is that consumers could learn distressing health information or upsetting information about family relationships and secrets. An estimated 35%–40% of patients undergoing DTCGT may not consider the possibility of receiving unwanted or distressing results (Kilbride et al., 2018).

Pretest counseling with a genetics professional involves an extensive discussion of the risks, benefits, and limitations of testing. Genetics professionals will explain that through testing an individual could learn distressing information or long-held family secrets. This type of disclosure and warning is a major component of pretest counseling, as well as part of informed consent. During disclosure of potentially distressing results and information, the genetics professional can provide psychosocial support and help a patient to cope with distressing information. On the other hand, in DTCGT, the consumer can receive distressing information unfiltered and without any readily available support or resources to understand the information.

Most DTCGT companies do not sequence the entire genome. They typically use SNP genotyping, which checks for the presence or absence of specific variants throughout the genetic code, such as a particular single nucleotide (Horton et al., 2019). A customer may think that sequencing is comprehensive or that numerous genes have been tested; however, in reality, testing may only involve a few SNPs or specific variants known to be associated with a higher risk for developing a disease.

Because many DTCGT laboratories are not CLIA certified, concerns about the accuracy of the results have been raised. For this reason, DTCGT companies recommend that test results be confirmed in a CLIA-certified laboratory. Additionally, some of the test results are not actionable. Consumers may also act on testing results that may be inaccurate or incomplete, or they could misinterpret the test results. Some DTCGT companies provide resources and access to genetics professionals, as well as scientific and technological information about testing processes and procedures. Other companies are not as transparent. CLIA certification helps to assure consumers that proper laboratory processes are in place and that results have clinical validity. Testing companies may or may not disclose clinical utility. A content analysis of 23 health-related DTCGT websites found that information about the benefits of the testing outweighed information about its risks and limitations by a ratio of six benefits to one risk or potential limitation of testing (Phillips, 2017).

A person's genetic data represent personal, private health information, and as a result, privacy of consumers choosing DTCGT is an important issue. Consumers should understand how the data are utilized after results are released. Usually, such information is contained in the fine print of the privacy statement that consumers agree to when they order testing. Many people who purchase testing never read the privacy statement or understand what rights they are signing away. For example, many of the DTCGT companies have the consumer agree to a terms of service agreement and privacy statement, both of which may be 25 pages or more in length (Artin et al., 2019). These legal documents allow the DTCGT company to utilize various types of personal information, including self-reported information, for research and to sell deidentified data as perpetual, royalty-free, worldwide, transferable licenses to pharmaceutical and other companies for research and product development. DTCGT may also utilize the extracted DNA for other types of research.

Although the Genetic Information Nondiscrimination Act (GINA) of 2008 provides federal protections against discrimination for employment and health insurance, consumers undergoing DTCGT might not fully understand the risks that disclosure of genetic results pose when they are trying to obtain life insurance, long-term care insurance, or disability insurance (Horton et al., 2019). In a clinical setting, during pretest genetic counseling, credentialed genetics professionals carefully review this information.

RAW DATA

Many DTCGT companies can provide consumers with the raw data that include extensive unanalyzed information about their genome. Genome sequencing is becoming more widely used in DTCGT genetic tests to identify the variants present within it. It is important to note that detecting variants is not the same as knowing and understanding the clinical significance of the variants (Horton et al., 2019).

Most companies caution the consumer that the raw data are only for research purposes and not to be used for diagnostic purposes. However, online services offer analysis and interpretation of the raw data collected by another company, for a fee. Regulation of these services is scarce. Third-party interpretation services can analyze the data and potentially provide the customer with more information about disease risk, traits, and ancestry. Depending on the quality of the interpretation, however, false positives and other errors can be reported, causing the consumer undue stress and anxiety. Errors occur because these services typically analyze the data by cross-referencing the data against freely available genetic databases, resulting in the construction of a report based on interpretations from these databases (Horton et al., 2019).

IMPLICATIONS FOR PRACTICE

Given the rising use of DTCGT, healthcare professionals should expect patients to present the results of these tests or arrive to appointments with questions about clinical genetic testing and DTCGT. Patients may also have questions regarding the data analysis in a DTCGT report or a third-party interpretation. When patients present with these types of results, they must be confirmed in a CLIA-certified laboratory (Artin et al., 2019).

Once patients have completed DTCGT, they are often unprepared for the consequences of testing, as in the case of a 46-year-old woman who requested testing for her daughter. The woman was divorced from and had little contact with her daughter's father. She purchased DTCGT for herself and her daughter for health and ancestry testing, intending it to be a fun Christmas gift. The daughter's report showed one of the *BRCA2* founder mutations, but it was not detected in the mother. A consultation with the mother outlined the complexities of this case. The daughter cannot consent, only assent, to confirmatory testing because she is younger than 18 years old. The daughter and mother were unprepared for these test results. The family history did not show any obvious signs that would have led to suspicion of hereditary breast and ovarian cancer syndrome.

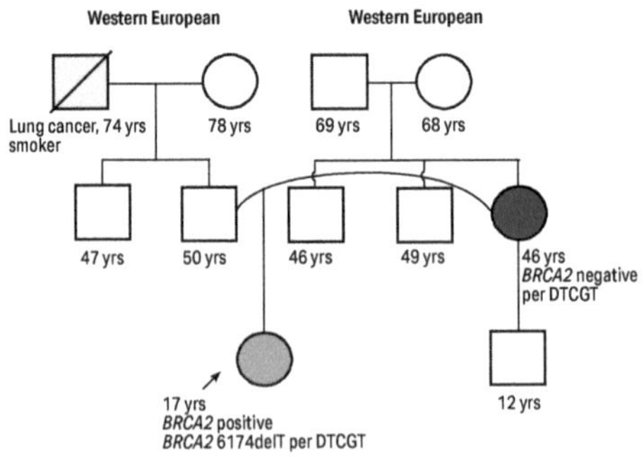

The daughter had not purchased life or disability insurance, and she was unsure of life past graduating from high school. The father was unwilling to engage in testing to better understand maternal or paternal transmission, and on further exploration, misattributed paternity was possible, suggesting that he is not the biologic father. If this family had engaged in pretest counseling, they would have been better prepared for the possibility of distressing results and complicated relationships. The effects on testing would have been discussed, including misattributed paternity. Testing would not have been offered to the daughter for adult-onset diseases, and the daughter would have been instructed to obtain adequate and appropriate life and disability insurance prior to testing. The mother is guilt-ridden and distressed over this Christmas gift gone wrong. This family could have avoided many of these problems if the mother had consulted with a genetics professional rather than using DTCGT.

During consultation, patients should be told that DTCGT is not diagnostic and provides very limited information on disease risk. Interpretation of genetic testing results can be complex and is best managed by a genetics professional (Schleit et al., 2019). Tests need to be interpreted in the context of information such as family and personal medical history and other risk factors.

In this exemplary case, a family had been receiving cancer genetic counseling and education, and the proband, a 41-year-old woman with a history of breast cancer, was known to carry the common founder *CHEK2* c.1100delC mutation. The woman wanted her mother to be tested for this mutation. The father had been tested and did not carry it. Given the family history and genetic testing to date, the mother was an obligate carrier.

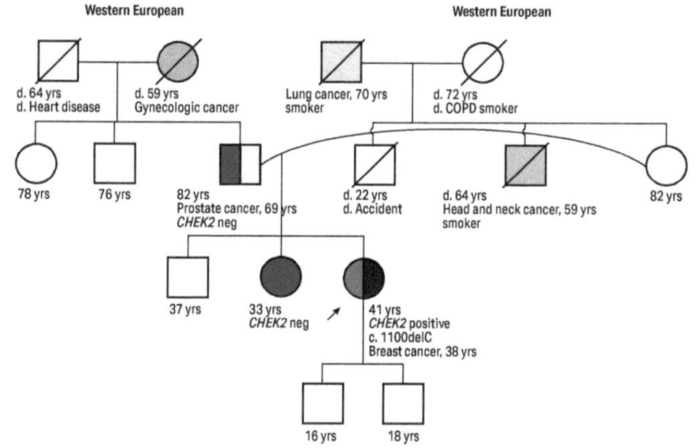

The mother was 82 years old and had multiple medical issues. She was not willing to engage in more aggressive screening or preventive surgery regardless of the outcome of the testing. She was insured through Medicare, which would not cover the costs of testing because she did not have a cancer diagnosis and it was not going to change her management. The family was offered the option of paying for the testing out of pocket and the alternative of not testing, assuming the mother carried the pathogenic variant. The family thought the costs were too high. A week later the daughter called and stated she had figured out how to get her mother genetic testing at a significantly lower cost through the DTCGT 23andMe. Even though the family had a relatively common *CHEK2* mutation, it would not be detected by 23andMe. The daughter was adamant that this was a cost-effective means to get her mother tested and that the website said it offered a cancer genetic test for breast cancer. The genetic counselor instructed her to look more closely at what was tested, and the daughter found that *CHEK2* was not covered in the testing results. Ultimately, the family decided not to pursue testing in the mother and assume she is an obligate carrier.

Despite having had intensive and multiple genetic counseling sessions, this family thought that DTCGT would be a less costly, equivalent substitute. When patients see the words "genetic testing," they may assume it tests for all genetic conditions. It is essential for healthcare providers to point out the differences between diagnostic tests and DTCGT.

SUMMARY

Although DTCGT has become commonplace among the general public and means big business for the companies promoting and selling such testing, consumers may be misled by the results of unproven or invalid tests, as well as tests that have limited clinical utility. It is important to acknowledge that the DTCGT business has increased public awareness about the role of genomics in health and provides an opportunity for healthcare providers to educate individuals about the importance of personal and medical family history in the selection of recommendations for care. Without guidance from a healthcare provider, consumers could be making important decisions about treatment or prevention based on inaccurate, incomplete, or misunderstood information about their health. For example, a woman who tests negative for the three founder *BRCA* mutations may mistakenly conclude that she does not have elevated risk for developing cancer when she actually harbors another breast cancer susceptibility gene that has implications for her health and health care, as well as that of her siblings, children, and other relatives. Conversely, an individual who has undergone testing may engage in inappropriate and potentially harmful health-related behaviors if the risk is overestimated.

Genetic testing provides only one piece of information about a person's health. Other genetic and environmental factors, lifestyle choices, and family medical history affect a person's risk of developing many disorders. These factors are discussed during a consultation with a physician or genetic counselor but, in many cases, are not addressed by DTCGT. Psychosocial distress for the individual and the family following DTCGT is another concern. Without genetic counseling prior to genetic testing, individuals may not be emotionally prepared to learn that they have increased risk for developing a disease for which there may or may not be a means to decrease or mitigate the risk, thus causing increased distress (Barton, 2017).

These risks and concerns are not always communicated to the customer by the testing company prior to purchasing a test. Also, detailed information about the privacy of the consumer's genetic data may only be found in the terms and conditions section and not highlighted on the main website pages.

When patients ask about DTCGT, nurses have a prime opportunity to discuss family history of malignancy and considerations regarding DTCGT. Formal genetic counseling with a credentialed genetics professional allows for selection of the most appropriate test; anticipatory guidance about the strengths, limitations, and risks of genetic testing; psychosocial support; and appropriate interpretation of the results. If patients inquire about DTCGT or raise other questions about genetic risk and healthcare providers ignore or discount these questions, patients may turn to DTCGT and run the risk of receiving distressing information or inappropriate interpretation of results.

REFERENCES

Allyse, M.A., Robinson, D.H., Ferber, M.J., & Sharp, R.R. (2018). Direct-to-consumer testing 2.0: Emerging models of direct-to-consumer genetic testing. *Mayo Clinic Proceedings, 93*(1), 113–120. https://doi.org/10.1016/j.mayocp.2017.11.001

AP News. (2020, October 28). Global direct-to-consumer (DTC) genetic testing market to expand at about 14.9% CAGR during 2020–2026 – ZMR. https://apnews.com/press-release/marketersmedia/business-corporate-news-north-america-products-and-services-genetic-testing-2a8ee087dccb8c1efdf078596b341dbc

Artin, M.G., Stiles, D., Kiryluk, K., & Chung, W. (2019). Cases in precision medicine: When patients present with direct-to-consumer genetic test results. *Annals of Internal Medicine, 170*(9), 643–650. https://doi.org/10.7326/m18-2356

Barton, M.K. (2017). Health behaviors not significantly changed by direct-to-consumer genetic testing. *CA: A Cancer Journal for Clinicians, 67*(3), 175–176. https://doi.org/10.3322/caac.21368

Gill, J., Obley, A.J., & Prasad, V. (2018). Direct-to-consumer genetic testing: The implications of the US FDA's first marketing authorization for *BRCA* mutation testing. *JAMA, 319*(23), 2377–2378. https://doi.org/10.1001/jama.2018.5330

Horton, R., Crawford, G., Freeman, L., Fenwick, A., Wright, C.F., & Lucassen, A. (2019). Direct-to-consumer genetic testing. *BMJ, 367,* l5688. https://doi.org/10.1136/bmj.l5688

Khan, R., & Mittelman, D. (2018). Consumer genomics will change your life, whether you get tested or not. *Genome Biology, 19,* 120. https://doi.org/10.1186/s13059-018-1506-1

Kilbride, M.K., Domchek, S.M., & Bradbury, A.R. (2018). Ethical implications of direct-to-consumer hereditary cancer tests. *JAMA Oncology, 4*(10), 1327–1328. https://doi.org/10.1001/jamaoncol.2018.2439

Mahon, S.M. (2016). The deceptive appeal of direct-to-consumer genetics. *Annals of Internal Medicine, 165*(9), 675–676. https://doi.org/10.7326/L16-0333

Mahon, S.M. (2018). Direct-to-consumer genetic testing: Helping patients make informed choices. *Clinical Journal of Oncology Nursing, 22*(1), 33–36. https://doi.org/10.1188/18.CJON.33-36

Phillips, A.M. (2017). Reading the fine print when buying your genetic self online: Direct-to-consumer genetic testing terms and conditions. *New Genetics and Society, 36*(3), 273–295. https://doi.org/10.1080/14636778.2017.1352468

Ramos, E., & Weissman, S.M. (2018). The dawn of consumer-directed testing. *American Journal of Medical Genetics Part C: Seminars in Medical Genetics, 178*(1), 89–97. https://doi.org/10.1002/ajmg.c.31603

Schleit, J., Naylor, L.V., & Hisama, F.M. (2019). First, do no harm: Direct-to-consumer genetic testing. *Genetics in Medicine, 21*(2), 510–511. https://doi.org/10.1038/s41436-018-0071-z

Stoeklé, H.-C., Mamzer-Bruneel, M.-F., Vogt, G., & Hervé, C. (2016). 23andMe: A new two-sided data-banking market model. *BMC Medical Ethics, 17,* 19. https://doi.org/10.1186/s12910-016-0101-9

Wynn, J., & Chung, W.K. (2017). 23andMe paves the way for direct-to-consumer genetic health risk tests of limited clinical utility. *Annals of Internal Medicine, 167*(2), 125–126. https://doi.org/10.7326/M17-1045

CHAPTER 5

Risks and Management Recommendations for Specific Hereditary Cancer Syndromes

INTRODUCTION

One goal of genetic testing is to identify individuals with known germline risk and develop a plan to manage the increased risk of developing cancer. Management of cancer risk may include more intensive or more frequent screening (often at a younger age than recommended in the general population), risk-reducing surgery, and chemoprevention. The importance of an accurate family medical history when making these recommendations cannot be overemphasized. The presentation of malignancies in a family and ages at onset also influence when and how recommendations will be implemented.

Recommendations for management of germline pathogenic variants is continually evolving. The information presented in this chapter is based on the available evidence-based recommendations at the time of this writing. Most genetics professionals will provide, in addition to a copy of the test results, a letter or summary of recommended management.

During a patient care visit with an individual who has seen a genetics professional and has received genetic testing results showing a pathogenic variant, a negative result, or an indeterminate result, nurses should anticipate that the patient will have been given recommendations for care. Nurses then must ensure that these recommendations are implemented. These recommendations for care should be reviewed with a genetics professional every 12–18 months to ascertain that they are still current.

Nurses should be aware of resources for information about management of germline risk. The National Comprehensive Cancer Network publishes guidelines for management in those with germline risk for breast, ovarian, prostate, and pancreatic cancer syndromes and colon cancers syndromes, available at www.nccn.org.

These guidelines are updated on a regular basis. *GeneReviews*® (www.ncbi.nlm.nih.gov/books/NBK1116) is an online resource published by the University of Washington that contains chapters on germline syndromes and includes extensive information on hereditary risk, such as epidemiologic information, associated risks, testing strategies, and recommendations for care. Experts write these chapters and review and update them on a regular basis. For some of the less common syndromes, specialty organizations dedicated to the study, care, and treatment of these syndromes issue recommendations for care. Genetics professionals can utilize all of these resources when making recommendations for care.

This chapter summarizes many of the more commonly seen hereditary cancer syndromes. Each description includes information about the gene(s) associated with the syndrome, known risks and the magnitude of risk (when available), recommended screening and prevention strategies, any other unique information about the hereditary cancer syndrome, and the age to test individuals. This general information will be helpful to nurses so that they can reinforce to patients the information about cancer risk and the importance of testing in their family, as well as to ascertain whether recommendations for cancer prevention and early detection are performed.

People with known hereditary risk should also receive education and information on lifestyle behaviors that can further reduce the risk of developing cancer. This type of education should include information about the importance of avoiding tobacco use, reducing exposure to ultraviolet (UV) light, undergoing regular vaccination (including for human papillomavirus), adopting a low-fat/high-fiber diet, and engaging in regular exercise or physical activity. Although these behaviors will not completely eliminate cancer risk, these lifestyle behaviors can help to reduce cancer risk for all people, but especially so for those with increased genetic risk.

By providing education about risks and ensuring that recommendations for care are implemented, nurses can ultimately help to reduce the morbidity and mortality associated with hereditary cancer syndromes.

AIP

Cancer Risks

- Pathogenic variants in the *AIP* gene cause 15%–25% of cases of familial isolated pituitary adenoma. The most commonly occurring pituitary adenomas are growth hormone–secreting adenomas (somatotropinoma), followed by prolactin-secreting adenomas (prolactinoma), growth hormone and prolactin–cosecreting adenomas (somatomammotropinoma), and nonfunctioning pituitary adenomas.
- The risk of developing a pituitary tumor is approximately 15%–30%.
- Average age at onset of cancer is 18–34 years, and cancer is twice as common in males.

Management Options for Screening and Risk Reduction

Increased Screening: Adults

- Annual clinical assessment for symptoms, including amenorrhea, sexual problems, galactorrhea, infertility, visual field defects, and headaches
- Annual pituitary function tests (insulin-like growth factor 1, prolactin, estradiol/testosterone, luteinizing hormone, follicle-stimulating hormone, free thyroxine, morning cortisol)
- Pituitary magnetic resonance imaging (MRI) every five years if clinical findings and pituitary function tests remain normal. Healthcare providers can consider discontinuing monitoring at approximately age 50 years, after which the likelihood of developing new pituitary adenomas is low.
- Annual clinical monitoring of secondary complications of the pituitary adenoma and its treatment (e.g., diabetes mellitus, hypertension, osteoarthritis, hypogonadism, osteoporosis)

Increased Screening: Children

- Annual screening beginning at age four years
- Baseline pituitary MRI at approximately age 10 years
- Consideration of repeating pituitary MRI every five years if clinical and pituitary function tests remain normal
- Documentation of pubertal development (Tanner stages)
- Height and weight, with calculation of height velocity
- Pituitary function tests, as recommended for adults

Age to Test Relatives

- By age four years, when screening would begin for families with a known pathogenic variant

Reference

Korbonits, M., & Kumar, A.V. (2020). *AIP* familial isolated pituitary adenomas. In M.P. Adam, H.H. Ardinger, R.A. Pagon, & S.E. Wallace (Eds.), *GeneReviews*®. University of Washington. https://www.ncbi.nlm.nih.gov/books/NBK97965

ALK

Cancer Risks

- Risk of developing a neuroblastoma, ganglioneuroblastoma, and ganglioneuroma is approximately 57% in those with a pathogenic variant of *ALK*.
- Risk for neuroblastic tumor development is highest in infancy and decreases by late childhood, with 98% of neuroblastic tumors occurring by age 10 years.

- Individuals with a pathogenic variation of *ALK* tend to develop tumors at a younger age (average nine months) than those without genetic predisposition (two to three years).

Management Options for Screening and Risk Reduction

Asymptomatic Children

- Physical examination, abdominal ultrasound examination, chest x-ray, and measurement of urine catecholamine metabolite levels (homovanillic acid and vanillylmandelic acid) every three months between birth and six years of age
- Physical examination, abdominal ultrasound examination, chest x-ray, and measurement of urine catecholamine metabolite levels (homovanillic acid and vanillylmandelic acid) every six months between age 6 and 10 years. Screening beyond age 10 years is not indicated.

After Successful Treatment of a Neuroblastic Tumor

- Continued screening for neuroblastoma. Children with *ALK*-related neuroblastoma are at risk for developing multiple primary tumors.
- Continued screening as described previously until 10 years of age

Age to Test Relatives

- As soon as possible at birth

Reference

Greengard, E.G., & Park, J.R. (2019). *ALK*-related neuroblastic tumor susceptibility. In M.P. Adam, H.H. Ardinger, R.A. Pagon, & S.E. Wallace (Eds.), *GeneReviews®*. University of Washington. https://www.ncbi.nlm.nih.gov/books/NBK24599

APC (*APC*-ASSOCIATED POLYPOSIS CONDITIONS: FAMILIAL ADENOMATOUS POLYPOSIS)

Cancer Risks

- People with a pathogenic variant of *APC* have a condition known as familial adenomatous polyposis (FAP) and develop hundreds to thousands of adenomatous colonic polyps beginning at age 16 years on average (range 7–36 years).
- By age 35 years, 95% of individuals with FAP have polyps. Without colectomy, risk of colon cancer is 100%.
- Mean age at colon cancer diagnosis in untreated individuals is 39 years (range 34–43 years).

- Extracolonic manifestations are variable and include polyps of the gastric fundus and duodenum (50%–90%), osteomas (20%), dental anomalies, congenital hypertrophy of the retinal pigment epithelium (75%), soft tissue tumors, desmoid tumors (20%–30%), and cribriform-morular variant of papillary thyroid cancer.
- Attenuated FAP is characterized by multiple colonic polyps (average of 30), more proximally located polyps, and a diagnosis of colon cancer at a later age than in FAP. Lifetime risk of colon cancer is 70%.

Management Options for Screening and Risk Reduction

Increased Screening

- Annual colonoscopy starting at age 10–12 years for FAP; colonoscopy every two to three years beginning in late teens for attenuated FAP. When adenomas are detected, colonoscopy with polypectomy should occur every one to two years depending on polyp burden.
- Esophagogastroduodenoscopy every six months to four years, depending on duodenal adenoma burden, starting at age 20–25 years. Surveillance should include complete visualization of the ampulla of Vater. The stomach should be visualized at the time of upper endoscopy.
- Annual physical examination, including evaluation for extraintestinal manifestations and neurologic deficits
- Annual thyroid examination starting in late teens. An annual thyroid ultrasound may be considered, with fine-needle aspiration if thyroid nodules are present.
- Annual abdominal palpation for desmoids. If a patient has a family history of desmoids, MRI or computed tomography (CT) scan should occur within 1–3 years after colectomy, then every 5–10 years. Data to support screening and treatment of desmoid tumors are limited.
- Addition of small bowel visualization to CT or MRI for desmoids (if applicable), especially for extensive duodenal polyposis (National Comprehensive Cancer Network recommendation)
- Following total colectomy, routine endoscopic surveillance of the ileal pouch every one to three years
- Following subtotal colectomy with ileorectal anastomosis, surveillance of the remaining rectum every 6–12 months, depending on the number of polyps
- Following total colectomy with end ileostomy, ileoscopy every two years. Evidence suggests that the risk of desmoid tumors is increased by abdominal surgery, and risk may be higher for surgical procedures that require two stages to complete. Individuals at high risk for desmoids (e.g., women, those with *APC* pathogenic variants in codons 1395–1493, those with a family history of desmoids) may consider delaying surgery longer than might otherwise be recommended or may consider undergoing a surgery that is likely to be definitive for colorectal cancer risk (e.g., total colectomy with ileostomy) in order to minimize the likelihood of a second surgery.

Risk-Reducing Surgery

- Diagnosis or suspicion of colorectal cancer and significant symptoms (e.g., bleeding, obstruction) are absolute indications for colectomy.
- Relative indications for colectomy include the following:
  - Presence of multiple adenomas larger than 6 mm that cannot be reasonably removed endoscopically
  - Significant increase in adenoma number between surveillance exams
  - Presence of adenomas with high-grade dysplasia
  - Inability to adequately survey the colon (e.g., innumerous diminutive adenomas, limited access to or compliance with colonoscopy)

Other Preventive Measures

- Several studies have shown that nonsteroidal anti-inflammatory drugs have caused regression of adenomas in FAP and decreased the polyp burden; however, no U.S. Food and Drug Administration–approved chemopreventive agents for FAP are currently available.

Age to Test Relatives

- Approximately age 10 years

References

Jasperson, K.W., Patel, S.G., & Ahnen, D.J. (2017). *APC*-associated polyposis conditions. In M.P. Adam, H.H. Ardinger, R.A. Pagon, & S.E. Wallace (Eds.), *GeneReviews®*. University of Washington. https://www.ncbi.nlm.nih.gov/books/NBK1345

National Comprehensive Cancer Network. (2020). *NCCN Clinical Practice Guidelines in Oncology (NCCN Guidelines®): Genetic/familial high-risk assessment: Colorectal* [v.1.2020]. https://www.nccn.org/professionals/physician_gls/pdf/genetics_colon.pdf

ATM

Cancer Risks

- Risk of breast cancer is estimated to be 17%–52% in women with an *ATM* pathogenic variant.
- Risk of colorectal cancer may be increased.
- Risk of ovarian cancer is potentially increased; risk is higher with a family history of ovarian cancer.
- Risk of pancreatic cancer is potentially increased; risk is higher with a family history of pancreatic cancer.
- Risk of prostate cancer is potentially increased; risk is higher with a family history of prostate cancer.

Management Options for Screening and Risk Reduction

Increased Screening

- Annual mammography beginning at age 30–40 years, depending on family history. Consideration can be given to adding breast MRI, alternating every six months with mammography.
- Clinical breast exam (ideally by a breast surgeon) every 6–12 months, starting at age 25 years
- Monthly breast self-examination starting at age 25 years, with prompt evaluation of any change
- Annual pelvic examination with careful attention to the ovaries. For those with a family history of ovarian cancer, special consideration can be given to annual transvaginal ultrasound screening of the ovaries, beginning at approximately age 30 years, until the patient is ready to consider surgical options.
- Colonoscopy every three to five years, starting at age 30 years (or earlier depending on family history). This should be performed more frequently if polyps are detected.
- Early prostate screening with a rectal exam of the prostate and a prostate-specific antigen (PSA) test, starting at age 40 years, especially in men with a family history of prostate cancer
- Annual pancreatic screening (men and women), starting at age 40 years or 10 years prior to the age of the youngest pancreatic cancer diagnosis in the family, with MRI/magnetic resonance cholangiopancreatography (MRCP), endoscopic ultrasound (EUS), fasting blood glucose, and glycated hemoglobin (HbA1c). Annual follow-up includes alternating MRI/MRCP and EUS with annual fasting blood glucose and HbA1c.

Risk-Reducing Surgery

- Bilateral risk-reducing mastectomy with an option of breast reconstruction. Surgery reduces the chance of developing breast cancer by at least 95%.
- Possible surgery to remove the ovaries and fallopian tubes at age 40–50 years, after childbearing, especially in women with a family history of ovarian cancer. Surgery reduces the risk of ovarian cancer by approximately 80%–90%.

Age to Test Relatives

- Approximately age 25 years
- People with two pathogenic copies of *ATM* are at risk for an autosomal dominant condition known as ataxia telangiectasia. Carriers may benefit from preconception genetic counseling and testing.

References

Goggins, M., Overbeek, K.A., Brand, R., Syngal, S., Del Chiaro, M., Bartsch, D.K., ... Bruno, M. (2019). Management of patients with increased risk for familial pancreatic cancer: Updated recommendations from the International Cancer of the Pancreas Screening (CAPS) Consortium. *Gut, 69*(1), 7–17. https://doi.org/10.1136/gutjnl-2019-319352

National Comprehensive Cancer Network. (2020a). *NCCN Clinical Practice Guidelines in Oncology (NCCN Guidelines®): Genetic/familial high-risk assessment: Breast, ovarian, and pancreatic* [v.2.2021]. https://www.nccn.org/professionals/physician_gls/pdf/genetics_bop.pdf
National Comprehensive Cancer Network. (2020b). *NCCN Clinical Practice Guidelines in Oncology (NCCN Guidelines®): Genetic/familial high-risk assessment: Colorectal* [v.1.2020]. https://www.nccn.org/professionals/physician_gls/pdf/genetics_colon.pdf

AXIN2

Cancer Risks

- People with an *AXIN2* pathogenic variant have an increased risk of colon polyps. Cases of early onset (before age 45 years) have been reported, but the exact risk is unknown.
- Oligodontia is the rare congenital absence of more than six teeth in primary and/or permanent teeth that has been seen in individuals with pathogenic variants in *AXIN2*.
- A few cases of early-onset breast cancer have been reported in families with *AXIN2* pathogenic variants.

Management Options for Screening and Risk Reduction

Increased Screening

- Colonoscopy every one to two years, depending on whether polyps are detected, starting at age 25–30 years
- Annual clinical breast exam, starting at age 25 years
- Monthly breast self-examination starting at age 18 years, with prompt evaluation of any change
- Annual mammography, starting at age 40 years; earlier for a history of breast cancer in the family

Risk-Reducing Surgery

- Consideration of colectomy if polyp burden becomes too high to manage with regular colonoscopy

Age to Test Relatives

- Approximately age 25 years

References

National Comprehensive Cancer Network. (2020). *NCCN Clinical Practice Guidelines in Oncology (NCCN Guidelines®): Genetic/familial high-risk assessment: Colorectal* [v.1.2020]. https://www.nccn.org/professionals/physician_gls/pdf/genetics_colon.pdf
U.S. National Library of Medicine. (2021). *AXIN2*. In *Gene*. https://www.ncbi.nlm.nih.gov/gene/8313

BAP1

Cancer Risks

- Atypical Spitz tumors may be the most common manifestation of a *BAP1* pathogenic variant.
- Median age at onset of uveal melanoma, the most common cancer in people with a *BAP1* pathogenic variant, is 51 years, which is younger than the onset in the general population (62 years). The tumors are generally more aggressive, with higher risk for metastasis and reduced survival.
- Median age at onset of mesothelioma in individuals with a *BAP1* pathogenic variant is earlier (55–58 years) than that of sporadic mesothelioma (62–68 years). Of cases related to *BAP1* pathogenic variants, 80% are pleural mesothelioma and 20% are peritoneal mesothelioma.
- Cutaneous melanoma is the third most common cancer in people with a *BAP1* pathogenic variant.
- Risk of renal cell cancer is higher and tends to occur at younger age (mean age 47 years; 64 years in the general population).
- People with a *BAP1* pathogenic variant may also have multiple basal cell skin cancers.
- Other cancers that may be associated with *BAP1* pathogenic variants include breast cancer, cholangiocarcinoma, meningioma, neuroendocrine tumors, non-small cell lung adenocarcinoma, and thyroid cancer, but the risk is not understood.

Management Options for Screening and Risk Reduction

Increased Screening

- Annual dilated eye examination and imaging by an ocular oncologist, beginning at approximately age 11 years. Examination should consist of direct and indirect ophthalmoscopy, fundus photography, and ocular ultrasound.
- No reliable early disease symptoms or screening modalities exist for mesothelioma. An annual evaluation is recommended for late manifestations of mesothelioma, which can include chest pain, cough, fever, shortness of breath, dysphagia, hoarseness, weight loss, fever, upper body and face edema, abdominal pain, ascites, nausea, vomiting, and constipation. An annual physical examination is recommended to look for signs of pleurisy, peritonitis, ascites, and pleural effusion.
- Abdominal MRI and urinalysis every two years, for clear cell renal carcinoma. Evaluation of the peritoneum and pleura can also be considered.
- Annual abdominal ultrasound examination
- Annual full body dermatologic examination, beginning at approximately age 12 years

Other Preventive Measures

- Arc welding has been associated with risk of uveal melanoma and should be avoided if possible.

- Sunglasses with high UVA and UVB protection can reduce risk of cancer on the eyelids, but data regarding the benefit of sunglasses for uveal melanoma are lacking.
- Asbestos exposure and tobacco use should be avoided.
- Primary prevention is limited to measures typically used to reduce the risk of cutaneous melanoma, including limiting sun exposure, using sunscreen with SPF 30 or higher, and wearing protective clothing, including hats.

Age to Test Relatives

- Approximately age 10 years

References

Pilarski, R., Rai, K., Cebulla, C., & Abdel-Rahman, M. (2020) *BAP1* tumor predisposition syndrome. In M.P. Adam, H.H. Ardinger, R.A. Pagon, & S.E. Wallace (Eds.), *GeneReviews®*. University of Washington. https://www.ncbi.nlm.nih.gov/books/NBK390611

Star, P., Goodwin, A., Kapoor, R., Conway, R.M., Long, G.V., Scolyer, R.A., & Guitera, P. (2018). Germline *BAP1*-positive patients: The dilemmas of cancer surveillance and a proposed interdisciplinary consensus monitoring strategy. *European Journal of Cancer, 92*, 48–53. https://doi.org/10.1016/j.ejca.2017.12.022

BARD1

Cancer Risks

- Women with a *BARD1* pathogenic variant have an increased risk for developing breast cancer, especially triple-negative breast cancer. Risk is estimated to be two to three times the general population (lifetime risk 25%–40%).
- Risks of ovarian, pancreatic, and prostate cancer may be increased.

Management Options for Screening and Risk Reduction

Increased Screening

- Annual breast MRI (or mammography if MRI is unavailable), beginning at age 25–29 years depending on family history (early-onset breast cancer). At age 30 years and beyond, both annual mammography and breast MRI are recommended, alternating every six months, depending on family history.
- Clinical breast exam (ideally by a breast surgeon) every 6–12 months, starting at age 25 years
- Monthly breast self-examination starting at age 18 years, with prompt evaluation of any change
- Careful gynecologic examination annually, with attention to the ovaries. Pelvic ultrasound can be considered for patients with a family history of ovarian cancer.

Risk-Reducing Surgery

- Bilateral risk-reducing mastectomy with an option of breast reconstruction in women with a significant family history of breast cancer. This type of surgery reduces the chance of developing breast cancer by at least 95%.

Age to Test Relatives

- Approximately age 25 years

References

National Comprehensive Cancer Network. (2020). *NCCN Clinical Practice Guidelines in Oncology (NCCN Guidelines®): Genetic/familial high-risk assessment: Breast, ovarian, and pancreatic* [v.2.2021]. https://www.nccn.org/professionals/physician_gls/pdf/genetics_bop.pdf

Petrucelli, N., Daly, M.B., & Pal, T. (2016). *BRCA1*- and *BRCA2*-associated hereditary breast and ovarian cancer. In M.P. Adam, H.H. Ardinger, R.A. Pagon, & S.E. Wallace (Eds.), *GeneReviews®*. University of Washington. https://www.ncbi.nlm.nih.gov/books/NBK1247

BMPR1A

Cancer Risks

- People with pathogenic variants of *BMPR1A* are at risk for developing hamartomatous polyps.
- The incidence of colorectal cancer is 17%–22% by age 35 years and approaches 68% by age 60 years. The median age at diagnosis is 42 years.
- The incidence of gastric cancer is 21% in those with gastric polyps.
- Risk of pancreatic and small bowel cancer may be increased.

Management Options for Screening and Risk Reduction

Increased Screening

- Monitoring for rectal bleeding and anemia, abdominal pain, constipation, and diarrhea; screening by complete blood count starting by age 10 years
- Colonoscopy and upper endoscopy, starting at approximately age 15 years or earlier if symptoms occur. If no polyps are detected, screening should be repeated in two to three years. Once polyps are detected, annual screening is indicated.
- Consideration of capsule endoscopy to evaluate for small bowel cancer, starting at approximately age 15 years
- Annual pancreatic screening in people with a family history of pancreatic cancer, starting at age 40 years or 10 years prior to the age of the youngest pancreatic cancer diagnosis in the family, with MRI/MRCP, EUS, fasting blood glu-

cose, and HbA1c. Annual recommended follow-up includes alternating MRI/MRCP and EUS with annual fasting blood glucose and HbA1c.

Risk-Reducing Surgery

- Consideration of colectomy if there is an increase in polyps between screenings or malignancy is diagnosed

Age to Test Relatives

- Approximately age 5–10 years

References

Goggins, M., Overbeek, K.A., Brand, R., Syngal, S., Del Chiaro, M., Bartsch, D.K., ... Bruno, M. (2020). Management of patients with increased risk for familial pancreatic cancer: Updated recommendations from the International Cancer of the Pancreas Screening (CAPS) Consortium. *Gut, 69*(1), 7–17. https://doi.org/10.1136/gutjnl-2019-319352

Haidle, J.L., & Howe, J.R. (2017). Juvenile polyposis syndrome. In M.P. Adam, H.H. Ardinger, R.A. Pagon, & S.E. Wallace (Eds.), *GeneReviews®*. University of Washington. https://www.ncbi.nlm.nih.gov/books/NBK1469

National Comprehensive Cancer Network. (2020). *NCCN Clinical Practice Guidelines in Oncology (NCCN Guidelines®): Genetic/familial high-risk assessment: Colorectal* [v.1.2020]. https://www.nccn.org/professionals/physician_gls/pdf/genetics_colon.pdf

BRCA1 AND *BRCA2*

Cancer Risks

- Women with *BRCA1* or *BRCA2* pathogenic variants have a 38%–84% chance of developing breast cancer (12% in the general population).
- Women have a 10.8% increased risk of a second primary breast cancer within 10 years of first diagnosis or 62% by age 70 (2% within 5 years in the general population).
- The lifetime risk of developing ovarian cancer is 16%–27% with *BRCA1* or *BRCA2* pathogenic variants (1%–2% in the general population).
- Men with *BRCA2* pathogenic variants have an 8.9% lifetime risk for male breast cancer (less than 1% in the general population).
- Men with *BRCA1* or *BRCA2* pathogenic variants have a 20%–34% lifetime risk for prostate cancer (12% in the general population).
- Men and women have up to a 7% lifetime risk for pancreatic cancer (0.5% in the general population).
- For both men and women, there is an increased risk for developing melanoma.
- Fanconi anemia is associated with having two copies of a *BRCA2* pathogenic variant (one from each parent). The chance of having a child with Fanconi anemia is 25% for every pregnancy if both parents have a pathogenic variant.

Management Options for Screening and Risk Reduction

Increased Screening

- Annual breast MRI (or mammography if MRI is unavailable), beginning at age 25–29 years depending on family history. At age 30 years and beyond, annual mammography and breast MRI are recommended, alternating every six months, depending on family history.
- Clinical breast exam (ideally by a breast surgeon) every 6–12 months, starting at age 25 years
- Monthly breast self-examination starting at age 18 years, with prompt evaluation of any change
- Transvaginal ultrasound screening of the ovaries and a cancer antigen 125 (CA-125) blood test performed every six months, starting at age 30 years, until the patient is ready to consider surgical options
- In men, regular breast self-examination and annual clinical breast exam by a healthcare provider, starting at age 25 years
- Early prostate screening with a rectal exam of the prostate and a PSA blood test starting at age 40 years
- In men and women, full body skin examination for melanoma screening, with the frequency dependent on personal and family history of melanoma and atypical moles. Individuals should perform a monthly self-examination of the skin.
- In men and women, annual pancreatic screening starting at age 40 years or 10 years prior to the age of the youngest pancreatic cancer diagnosis in the family, with MRI/MRCP, EUS, fasting blood glucose, and HbA1c. Annual recommended follow-up includes alternating MRI/MRCP and EUS with annual fasting blood glucose and HbA1c.

Risk-Reducing Surgery

- Bilateral risk-reducing mastectomy with an option of breast reconstruction. Surgery reduces the chance of developing breast cancer by at least 95%.
- Surgery to remove the ovaries and fallopian tubes at age 35–45 years, when childbearing is complete. Surgery reduces the risk of ovarian cancer by approximately 80%–90%. If surgery occurs before natural menopause, it can reduce the risk of breast cancer by up to 50%.

Other Preventive Measures

- Tamoxifen and raloxifene, medications used to treat breast cancer, have been shown to reduce the risk of certain types of breast cancer by up to 50%. Individuals can consider using these drugs for five years.
- Hormonal contraceptive pills may also be considered following risk-reducing mastectomies to reduce the risk of ovarian cancer by up to 60%.
- Individuals should avoid artificial tanning.

- When in the sun, individuals should avoid sunburns by using broad-spectrum (UVA/UVB) sunscreen of SPF 30 or higher, seeking shade, covering up with clothing (including hats), and wearing UV-blocking sunglasses.

Age to Test Relatives

- Approximately age 25 years

References

Goggins, M., Overbeek, K.A., Brand, R., Syngal, S., Del Chiaro, M., Bartsch, D.K., ... Bruno, M. (2020). Management of patients with increased risk for familial pancreatic cancer: Updated recommendations from the International Cancer of the Pancreas Screening (CAPS) Consortium. *Gut, 69*(1), 7–17. https://doi.org/10.1136/gutjnl-2019-319352

National Comprehensive Cancer Network. (2020). *NCCN Clinical Practice Guidelines in Oncology (NCCN Guidelines®): Genetic/familial high-risk assessment: Breast, ovarian, and pancreatic* [v.2.2021]. https://www.nccn.org/professionals/physician_gls/pdf/genetics_bop.pdf

Petrucelli, N., Daly, M.B., & Pal, T. (2016). *BRCA1*- and *BRCA2*-associated hereditary breast and ovarian cancer. In M.P. Adam, H.H. Ardinger, R.A. Pagon, & S.E. Wallace (Eds.), *GeneReviews®*. University of Washington. https://www.ncbi.nlm.nih.gov/books/NBK1247

BRIP1

Cancer Risks

- With a *BRIP1* pathogenic variant, risk for ovarian cancer is increased, and it may be as high as 25% over a lifetime.
- Women may have an increased risk for developing breast cancer, although the exact risk is unknown.
- Fanconi anemia is associated with having two copies of a *BRIP1* pathogenic variant (one from each parent). The chance of having a child with Fanconi anemia is 25% for every pregnancy if both parents have a pathogenic variant.

Management Options for Screening and Risk Reduction

Increased Screening

- Transvaginal ultrasound screening of the ovaries and a CA-125 blood test performed every 6–12 months, beginning at approximately age 30 years, until the patient is ready to consider surgical options
- Depending on family history, consideration of breast MRI and mammography beginning as early as age 30 years
- Clinical breast exam (ideally by a breast surgeon) every 6–12 months, starting at age 25–30 years

- Monthly breast self-examination starting at age 18 years, with prompt evaluation of any change

Risk-Reducing Surgery
- Surgical removal of the ovaries and fallopian tubes, at age 45–50 years, when childbearing is complete
- Consideration of risk-reducing mastectomies for women with a significant family history of breast cancer

Age to Test Relatives
- Approximately age 25 years

Reference

National Comprehensive Cancer Network. (2020a). *NCCN Clinical Practice Guidelines in Oncology (NCCN Guidelines®): Genetic/familial high-risk assessment: Breast, ovarian, and pancreatic* [v.2.2021]. https://www.nccn.org/professionals/physician_gls/pdf/genetics_bop.pdf

CDC73

Cancer Risks

- Pathogenic variants in *CDC73* are associated with hyperparathyroidism-jaw tumor (HPT-JT) syndrome. Primary hyperparathyroidism, the main finding of HPT-JT syndrome, occurs in up to 95% of affected individuals. Onset is typically in late adolescence or early adulthood.
- In approximately 10%–15% of individuals with HPT-JT syndrome, primary hyperparathyroidism is caused by parathyroid carcinoma.
- Ossifying fibromas of the mandible or maxilla occur in 30%–40% of individuals with HPT-JT syndrome.
- Approximately 20% of individuals with HPT-JT syndrome have kidney lesions, most commonly cysts, and renal hamartomas. Wilms tumor is a rare occurrence.
- Benign and malignant uterine tumors occur more in women with HPT-JT syndrome.

Management Options for Screening and Risk Reduction

Increased Screening
- Annual measurement of serum calcium, intact parathyroid hormone, and 25-hydroxyvitamin D_3 levels, starting at age five years

- Periodic parathyroid ultrasound examination for the detection of nonfunctioning parathyroid carcinoma
- Dental panoramic x-ray with neck shielding at least every five years, starting at age 10 years
- Renal ultrasound examination at least every five years, starting at age 15 years
- For women, lifelong monitoring for uterine tumors with annual routine gynecologic exam and pelvic ultrasound examination, starting at age 25 years

Other Preventive Measures
- Dehydration should be avoided because it can lead to increased calcium levels and mental status changes.
- Radiation exposure should be minimized as much as possible.
- Biopsy of extrathyroidal tissue in the neck, which increases the risk of seeding of parathyroid tissue, should be avoided.

Age to Test Relatives
- Approximately age five years

References

Hyde, S.M., Rich, T.A., Waguespack, S.G., Perrier, N.D., & Hu, M.I. (2018). *CDC73*-related disorders. In M.P. Adam, H.H. Ardinger, R.A. Pagon, & S.E. Wallace (Eds.), *GeneReviews®*. University of Washington. https://www.ncbi.nlm.nih.gov/books/NBK3789

CDH1

Cancer Risks

- *CDH1* is associated with hereditary diffuse gastric cancer (HDGC), a poorly differentiated adenocarcinoma that infiltrates into the stomach wall, causing thickening of the wall without forming a distinct mass (signet ring carcinoma or isolated cell-type carcinoma). The average age at onset of HDGC is 38 years (range 14–69 years). Most cancers occur before age 40 years.
- The cumulative risk of gastric cancer by age 80 years is 70% for men and 56% for women.
- Women also have a 42% risk for lobular breast cancer. Average age at onset is 53 years.
- Risk for colorectal cancer may be increased, especially in families with a history of colorectal cancer.

Management Options for Screening and Risk Reduction

Increased Screening

- For at-risk individuals not ready to undergo risk-reducing total gastrectomy, screening with Cambridge protocol, a detailed 30-minute upper endoscopy every 6–12 months with multiple random biopsies and biopsies of subtle lesions, with screening beginning 5–10 years prior to the age of the youngest cancer diagnosis in the family
- Annual breast MRI (or mammography if MRI is unavailable), starting at age 25–29, years. At age 30 and beyond, annual mammography and breast MRI are recommended, alternating every six months.
- Clinical breast exam (ideally by a breast surgeon) every 6–12 months, starting at age 25 years
- Monthly breast self-examination starting at age 18 years, with prompt evaluation of any change
- Colonoscopy every three to five years, beginning at age 40 years or 10 years prior to the youngest age at diagnosis of colon cancer in families with histories of both HDGC and colon cancer

Risk-Reducing Surgery

- Prophylactic total gastrectomy (PTG) is recommended, rather than endoscopic surveillance. In individuals with a germline *CDH1* pathogenic variant who underwent PTG, early gastric cancers have been observed that were not detectable on endoscopy. Controversy has arisen related to this recommendation in how to manage families without a diagnosis of gastric cancer. Consideration needs to be given to family history, as PTG is associated with morbidity.
- Prophylactic mastectomy is not routinely recommended, but it may be a reasonable option for some women with an extensive family history of breast cancer, especially with diagnoses before age 45 years.

Age to Test Relatives

- Approximately age 16 years

References

Kaurah, P., & Huntsman, D.G. (2018). Hereditary diffuse gastric cancer. In M.P. Adam, H.H. Ardinger, R.A. Pagon, & S.E. Wallace (Eds.), *GeneReviews®*. University of Washington. https://www.ncbi.nlm.nih.gov/books/NBK1139

National Comprehensive Cancer Network. (2020). *NCCN Clinical Practice Guidelines in Oncology (NCCN Guidelines®): Genetic/familial high-risk assessment: Breast, ovarian, and pancreatic* [v.2.2021]. https://www.nccn.org/professionals/physician_gls/pdf/genetics_bop.pdf

Roberts, M.E., Ranola, J.M.O., Marshall, M.L., Susswein, L.R., Graceffo, S., Bohnert, K., ... Shirts, B.H. (2019). Comparison of *CDH1* penetrance estimates in clinically ascertained families vs families ascertained for multiple gastric cancers. *JAMA Oncology, 5*(9), 1325–1331. https://doi.org/10.1001/jamaoncol.2019.1208

van der Post, R.S., Vogelaar, I.P., Carneiro, F., Guilford, P., Huntsman, D., Hoogerbrugge, N., ... Bardram, L. (2015). Hereditary diffuse gastric cancer: Updated clinical guidelines with an emphasis on germline *CDH1* mutation carriers. *Journal of Medical Genetics, 52*(6), 361–374. https://doi.org/10.1136/jmedgenet-2015-103094

CDK4

Cancer Risks

- For people with a *CDK4* pathogenic variant, the risk for pancreatic cancer is increased.
- For people with a *CDK4* pathogenic variant, the risk for melanoma is increased, approaching 25%–75% by age 80 years.

Management Options for Screening and Risk Reduction

Increased Screening

- Full body skin examination for melanoma screening, with frequency depending on personal and family history of melanoma and atypical moles. Screening should be conducted at least annually. Whole-body skin photography may be helpful in individuals with many moles.
- Monthly self-examination of the skin
- For people with a family history of pancreatic cancer, annual pancreatic screening starting at age 40 years or 10 years prior to the age of the youngest pancreatic cancer diagnosis in the family, with MRI/MRCP, EUS, fasting blood glucose, and HbA1c. Annual recommended follow-up includes alternating MRI/MRCP and EUS with annual fasting blood glucose and HbA1c.

Risk-Reducing Surgery

- No recommendations

Other Preventive Measures

- Individuals should avoid artificial tanning.
- When in the sun, individuals should avoid sunburns by using a broad-spectrum (UVA/UVB) sunscreen with SPF 30 or higher, seeking shade, covering up with clothing (including hats), and wearing UV-blocking sunglasses.

Age to Test Relatives

- Approximately age 25 years

References

Goggins, M., Overbeek, K.A., Brand, R., Syngal, S., Del Chiaro, M., Bartsch, D.K., ... Bruno, M. (2020). Management of patients with increased risk for familial pancreatic cancer: Updated recommendations from the International Cancer of the Pancreas Screening (CAPS) Consortium. *Gut, 69*(1), 7–17. https://doi.org/10.1136/gutjnl-2019-319352

Read, J., Wadt, K.A.W., & Hayward, N.K. (2016). Melanoma genetics. *Journal of Medical Genetics, 53*(1), 1–14. https://doi.org/10.1136/jmedgenet-2015-103150

CDKN1B AND *CDKN2A*

Cancer Risks

- *CDKN1B* and *CDKN2A* pathogenic variants impose an increased risk of pancreatic cancer.
- Risk of melanoma is increased. Risk may approach 25%–75% by age 80 years.
- *CDNK1B* pathogenic variants have been associated with tumors (benign and malignant) in the pituitary glands.
- Risk of breast cancer may be increased in some *CDKN2A* pathogenic variants.

Management Options for Screening and Risk Reduction

Increased Screening

- Full body skin examination for melanoma screening, with the frequency depending on personal and family history of melanoma and atypical moles. Screening should be conducted at least annually. Whole-body skin photography may be helpful in individuals with many moles.
- Monthly self-examination of the skin
- For people with a family history of pancreatic cancer, annual pancreatic screening starting at age 40 years or 10 years prior to the age of the youngest pancreatic cancer diagnosis in the family, with MRI/MRCP, EUS, fasting blood glucose, and HbA1c. Annual recommended follow-up includes alternating MRI/MRCP and EUS with annual fasting blood glucose and HbA1c.
- Breast MRI and/or mammography at a younger age, with a family history of breast cancer
- Clinical breast exam (ideally by a breast surgeon) every 6–12 months, starting at age 25–30 years
- Monthly breast self-examination starting at age 18 years, with prompt evaluation of any change
- For family history of endocrine cancers, referral to an endocrinologist for yearly evaluation

Risk-Reducing Surgery

- No recommendations

Other Preventive Measures

- Individuals should avoid artificial tanning.
- When in the sun, individuals should avoid sunburns by using broad-spectrum (UVA/UVB) sunscreen of SPF 30 or higher, seeking shade, covering up with clothing (including hats), and wearing UV-blocking sunglasses.

Age to Test Relatives

- Approximately age 25 years

References

Goggins, M., Overbeek, K.A., Brand, R., Syngal, S., Del Chiaro, M., Bartsch, D.K., ... Bruno, M. (2020). Management of patients with increased risk for familial pancreatic cancer: Updated recommendations from the International Cancer of the Pancreas Screening (CAPS) Consortium. *Gut, 69*(1), 7–17. https://doi.org/10.1136/gutjnl-2019-319352

Read, J., Wadt, K.A.W., & Hayward, N.K. (2016). Melanoma genetics. *Journal of Medical Genetics, 53*(1), 1–14. https://doi.org/10.1136/jmedgenet-2015-103150

CHEK2

Cancer Risks

- Women with a *CHEK2* pathogenic variant have a 29%–59% chance of developing breast cancer (12% in the general population).
- Women have increased risk for a second primary breast cancer of 29% within 10 years of first diagnosis. The risk in the general population is 4% within 5 years.
- Men and women have an increased risk of colon cancer.
- The lifetime risk of developing ovarian and endometrial cancer is possibly increased.
- For men, risk of male breast cancer is increased.
- For men, risk of prostate cancer is increased.
- Individuals with a pathogenic variant may possibly have an increased risk of renal, thyroid, pancreatic, and stomach cancers.

Management Options for Screening and Risk Reduction

Increased Screening

- Annual mammography, starting at age 30 years, with consideration of alternating every six months with breast MRI
- Clinical breast exam (ideally by a breast surgeon) every 6–12 months, starting at age 25 years

- Monthly breast self-examination starting at age 18 years, with prompt evaluation of any change
- Colonoscopy starting at age 35–40 years or 10 years prior to the age of the youngest colon cancer diagnosis in the family. Screening should be repeated every three to five years or more frequently if polyps are detected. Upper endoscopy can be considered.
- Careful pelvic exam annually, with consideration of transvaginal ultrasound screening of the ovaries and endometrium; kidney evaluation at the same time
- For men, regular breast self-examination and annual clinical breast exam by a healthcare provider, beginning at age 30 years
- Early prostate screening with a rectal exam of the prostate and a PSA blood test, starting at age 40–45 years
- For people with a family history of pancreatic cancer, annual pancreatic screening starting at age 40 years or 10 years prior to the age of the youngest pancreatic cancer diagnosis in the family, with MRI/MRCP, EUS, fasting blood glucose, and HbA1c. Annual recommended follow-up includes alternating MRI/MRCP and EUS with annual fasting blood glucose and HbA1c.
- Annual palpation of the thyroid, with ultrasound evaluation of any palpable nodules
- Consideration of annual ultrasound of the kidneys, especially in those with a family history of renal cancer

Risk-Reducing Surgery

- Consideration of bilateral risk-reducing mastectomy with an option of breast reconstruction in women with a family history of breast cancer. Surgery reduces the chance of developing breast cancer by at least 95%.
- Consideration of surgery to remove the uterus, ovaries, and fallopian tubes, especially in women with a family history of gynecologic cancer. Surgery should occur at age 40–50 years, when childbearing is complete.

Other Preventive Measures

- Tamoxifen and raloxifene, medications used to treat breast cancer, have been shown to reduce the risk of certain types of breast cancer by up to 50%. Individuals can consider using these medications for five years.

Age to Test Relatives

- Approximately age 25 years

References

Goggins, M., Overbeek, K.A., Brand, R., Syngal, S., Del Chiaro, M., Bartsch, D.K., ... Bruno, M. (2020). Management of patients with increased risk for familial pancreatic cancer: Updated recommendations from the International Cancer of the Pancreas Screening (CAPS) Consortium. *Gut, 69*(1), 7–17. https://doi.org/10.1136/gutjnl-2019-319352

National Comprehensive Cancer Network. (2020a). *NCCN Clinical Practice Guidelines in Oncology (NCCN Guidelines®): Genetic/familial high-risk assessment: Breast, ovarian, and pancreatic* [v.2.2021]. https://www.nccn.org/professionals/physician_gls/pdf/genetics_bop.pdf

National Comprehensive Cancer Network. (2020b). *NCCN Clinical Practice Guidelines in Oncology (NCCN Guidelines®): Genetic/familial high-risk assessment: Colorectal* [v.1.2020]. https://www.nccn.org/professionals/physician_gls/pdf/genetics_colon.pdf

Petrucelli, N., Daly, M.B., & Pal, T. (2016). *BRCA1*- and *BRCA2*-associated hereditary breast and ovarian cancer. In M.P. Adam, H.H. Ardinger, R.A. Pagon, & S.E. Wallace (Eds.), *GeneReviews®*. University of Washington. https://www.ncbi.nlm.nih.gov/books/NBK1247

DICER1

Cancer Risks

- Cancers associated with *DICER1* are rare tumors, which include the following:
  - Botryoid-type embryonal rhabdomyosarcoma
  - Ciliary body medulloepithelioma
  - Cystic nephroma, usually before age four years
  - Nasal chondromesenchymal hamartoma
  - Nodular hyperplasia of the thyroid
  - Ovarian sex-cord stromal tumors
  - Pineoblastoma
  - Pituitary blastoma
  - Pleuropulmonary blastoma, usually occurring at approximately age two years, with shortness of breath with or without pneumothorax

Management Options for Screening and Risk Reduction

Increased Screening

- Annual physical examination and targeted review of systems
- Examination of all females at any age, for signs and symptoms of precocious puberty or virilization and masses in the abdomen or pelvis. If any signs are detected, appropriate imaging and laboratory evaluations should be performed. Laboratory testing includes alpha-fetoprotein, beta-human chorionic gonadotropin, lactate dehydrogenase, inhibin A and B, estradiol, testosterone, CA-125, and serum electrolytes including calcium. No current recommendations are available for laboratory screening in the absence of a mass or clinical findings of sex hormone excess.
- Chest CT at 3–6 months of age. If results are normal, a second chest CT should be performed at age 2.5–3 years, and a chest x-ray should also be performed every six months until the child is 8 years old. Frequency then decreases to every 12 months until the child is 12 years old.

- Thyroid ultrasound by age eight years. If the initial ultrasound is normal, it should be repeated every two to three years, based on the results of the child's physical exam.
- For patients treated with chemotherapy for pleuropulmonary blastoma, annual thyroid ultrasound for the first five years after treatment. If the ultrasound is normal, it should be repeated every two to three years.
- Abdominal ultrasound every six months until age 8 years, then annually until age 12 years
- Pelvic ultrasound once or twice a year, starting in early childhood and continuing into adulthood (usually to age 40 years)
- Screening evaluation for other tumors is based on clinical signs and symptoms.
  - A brain MRI is performed if a child is experiencing headaches, vomiting, decreased or double vision, difficulty with upward gaze, or early puberty, as well as if the child is diagnosed with Cushing syndrome.
  - Head and neck imaging is performed if the child has nasal obstruction.

Risk-Reducing Surgery
- No recommendations

Age to Test Relatives
- At birth

References

Schultz, K.A.P., Stewart, D.R., Kamihara, J., Bauer, A.J., Merideth, M.A., Stratton, P., ... Hill, A.D. (2020). *DICER1* tumor predisposition. In M.P. Adam, H.H. Ardinger, R.A. Pagon, & S.E. Wallace (Eds.), *GeneReviews®*. University of Washington. https://www.ncbi.nlm.nih.gov/books/NBK196157

Schultz, K.A.P., Williams, G.M., Kamihara, J., Stewart, D.R., Harris, A.K., Bauer, A.J., ... Hill, D.A. (2018). *DICER1* and associated conditions: Identification of at-risk individuals and recommended surveillance strategies. *Clinical Cancer Research, 24*(10), 2251–2261. https://doi.org/10.1158/1078-0432.CCR-17-3089

EPCAM, MLH1, MSH2, MSH3, MSH6, AND *PMS2* (LYNCH SYNDROME)

Cancer Risks

- For individuals with a pathogenic variant associated with Lynch syndrome, risk of colorectal cancer is 52%–82%. Mean age at diagnosis is 44–61 years.
- Risk of endometrial cancer is 25%–60%. Mean age at diagnosis is 48–62 years.
- Risk of gastric cancer is 6%–13%. Mean age at diagnosis is 56 years.
- Risk of ovarian cancer is 4%–20%. Mean age at diagnosis is 42.5 years, and approximately 30% are diagnosed before age 40 years.

- Risk of small bowel cancer is 4%–12%. Mean age at diagnosis is 49 years.
- Risk of urinary tract cancer is 2%–25%. Mean age at diagnosis is 52–60 years.
- Risk of brain cancer is 1%–4%. Mean age at diagnosis is 50 years.
- Risk of hepatobiliary tract cancer is 2%–4%. Mean age at diagnosis is 54–57 years.
- Risk of sebaceous adenoma is 1%–9%.
- Risk of pancreatic cancer is 0.4%–4%.
- Risk of prostate cancer is 9%–30%.
- Risk of breast cancer in females is 17%–37%. Risk in the general population is 12%–13%.

Management Options for Screening and Risk Reduction

Increased Screening

- Colonoscopy with removal of precancerous polyps every 1–2 years beginning at age 20–25 years or 2–5 years prior to the age of the youngest colon cancer diagnosis in the family, whichever is earlier
- Consideration of upper endoscopy every 3–5 years beginning at age 30–35 years, particularly for individuals with a family history of gastric cancer and those of Asian ancestry. Biopsies should be evaluated for *Helicobacter pylori* infections so that appropriate treatment can be initiated.
- Consideration of annual urinalysis beginning at age 30–35 years
- Annual physical exam, including a neurologic evaluation, beginning at age 25–30 years. At the time of this writing, no recommendations are available for routine imaging to screen for brain tumors.
- Consideration of capsule endoscopy and small bowel enterography. At the time of this writing, no recommendations are available for routine use of these approaches for small bowel screening, but they may be helpful for evaluating symptomatic individuals.
- Annual breast MRI (or mammography if MRI is unavailable) beginning at age 30 years. At age 30 years and beyond, mammography and breast MRI can be considered, alternating every six months, especially for families with a history of breast cancer.
- Clinical breast exam (ideally by a breast surgeon) every 6–12 months starting at age 25 years
- Monthly breast self-examination starting at age 18 years, with prompt evaluation of any change
- Consideration of transvaginal ultrasound screening of the ovaries and a CA-125 blood test every six months, beginning at approximately age 30 years, until the patient is ready to consider surgical options
- Consideration of annual full body skin examination for sebaceous adenoma screening

- Monthly self-examination of the skin
- For people with a family history of pancreatic cancer, annual pancreatic screening, starting at age 40 years or 10 years prior to the age of the youngest pancreatic cancer diagnosis in the family, with MRI/MRCP, EUS, fasting blood glucose, and HbA1c. Annual recommended follow-up includes alternating MRI/MRCP and EUS with annual fasting blood glucose and HbA1c.
- Prostate screening, including digital rectal examination and PSA testing, beginning at approximately age 45 years or earlier, depending on family history

Risk-Reducing Surgery

- Surgery to remove the uterus, ovaries, and fallopian tubes is recommended at age 35–45 years, when childbearing is complete. Surgery reduces the risk of ovarian cancer by approximately 80%–90%. If performed before natural menopause, surgery can reduce the risk of breast cancer by up to 50%.

Other Preventive Measures

- Individuals should avoid tobacco use, as it increases risk of colorectal cancer in this population.
- Use of aspirin can be considered to reduce colorectal cancer risk.

Age to Test Relatives

- Approximately age 25 years

References

Goggins, M., Overbeek, K.A., Brand, R., Syngal, S., Del Chiaro, M., Bartsch, D.K., ... Bruno, M. (2020). Management of patients with increased risk for familial pancreatic cancer: Updated recommendations from the International Cancer of the Pancreas Screening (CAPS) Consortium. *Gut, 69*(1), 7–17. https://doi.org/10.1136/gutjnl-2019-319352

Kohlmann, W., & Gruber, S.B. (2018). Lynch syndrome. In M.P. Adam, H.H. Ardinger, R.A. Pagon, & S.E. Wallace (Eds.), *GeneReviews®*. University of Washington. https://www.ncbi.nlm.nih.gov/books/NBK1211

National Comprehensive Cancer Network. (2020a). *NCCN Clinical Practice Guidelines in Oncology (NCCN Guidelines®): Genetic/familial high-risk assessment: Breast, ovarian, and pancreatic* [v.2.2021]. https://www.nccn.org/professionals/physician_gls/pdf/genetics_bop.pdf

National Comprehensive Cancer Network. (2020b). *NCCN Clinical Practice Guidelines in Oncology (NCCN Guidelines®): Genetic/familial high-risk assessment: Colorectal* [v.1.2020]. https://www.nccn.org/professionals/physician_gls/pdf/genetics_colon.pdf

FANCC

Cancer Risks

- Risk of breast cancer is increased for women with a *FANCC* pathogenic variant.
- Risk of pancreatic cancer is increased.

- Fanconi anemia is associated with having two copies of an *FANCC* pathogenic variant (one from each parent). The chance of having a child with Fanconi anemia is 25% for every pregnancy if both parents have a pathogenic variant.

Management Options for Screening and Risk Reduction

Increased Screening

- Consideration of screening with mammography and/or breast MRI every 6–12 months
- Clinical breast exam (ideally by a breast surgeon) every 6–12 months starting at age 25 years
- Monthly breast self-examination starting at age 18 years, with prompt evaluation of any change
- For men and women with a family history of pancreatic cancer, annual pancreatic screening, starting at age 40 years or 10 years prior to the age of the youngest pancreatic cancer diagnosis in the family, with MRI/MRCP, EUS, fasting blood glucose, and HbA1c. Annual recommended follow-up includes alternating MRI/MRCP and EUS with annual fasting blood glucose and HbA1c.

Risk-Reducing Surgery

- No recommendations, unless there is a significant family history of breast cancer

Age to Test Relatives

- Approximately age 25 years

References

Goggins, M., Overbeek, K.A., Brand, R., Syngal, S., Del Chiaro, M., Bartsch, D.K., ... Bruno, M. (2020). Management of patients with increased risk for familial pancreatic cancer: Updated recommendations from the International Cancer of the Pancreas Screening (CAPS) Consortium. *Gut, 69*(1), 7–17. https://doi.org/10.1136/gutjnl-2019-319352

Mehta, P.A., & Tolar, J. (2018). Fanconi anemia. In M.P. Adam, H.H. Ardinger, R.A. Pagon, & S.E. Wallace (Eds.), *GeneReviews®*. University of Washington. https://www.ncbi.nlm.nih.gov/books/NBK1401

National Comprehensive Cancer Network. (2020b). *NCCN Clinical Practice Guidelines in Oncology (NCCN Guidelines®): Genetic/familial high-risk assessment: Breast, ovarian, and pancreatic* [v.2.2021]. https://www.nccn.org/professionals/physician_gls/pdf/genetics_bop.pdf

FH

Cancer Risks

- Individuals with an *FH* pathogenic variant are at increased risk for developing cutaneous leiomyomas, which increase in size and number with age and are

painful or sensitive to light, touch, and cold temperature. Mean age at diagnosis is 30 years (range 10–77 years).
- Women with an *FH* pathogenic variant are at increased risk for developing uterine fibroids, and onset occurs at a younger age than in women in the general population. Mean age at diagnosis is approximately 30 years (range 18–53 years).
- Women are at increased risk for developing uterine leiomyosarcoma.
- Men and women with a pathogenic variant are at increased risk for developing renal tumors that are typically unilateral and solitary.
- Men and women may be at increased risk for developing pheochromocytomas and paragangliomas, but the magnitude of the risk is not clear.

Management Options for Screening and Risk Reduction

Increased Screening
- Consideration of full body skin examination, with frequency dependent on personal and family history of cutaneous leiomyomas
- Monthly self-examination of the skin
- Annual gynecologic exam starting by age 20–25 years, to assess for the presence of and size of uterine fibroids
- Starting at age 8 years, renal screening with MRI and contrast with 1–3 mm slices through the kidney (preferred). CT with contrast is an alternative.
- For families with a history of pheochromocytomas and paragangliomas, consideration of screening protocol recommendation for people with an *SDH* pathogenic variant

Risk-Reducing Surgery
- No recommendations

Age to Test Relatives
- Approximately age 5 years

References

Kamihara, J., Schultz, K.A., & Rana, H. (2020). *FH* tumor predisposition syndrome. In M.P. Adam, H.H. Ardinger, R.A. Pagon, & S.E. Wallace (Eds.), *GeneReviews®*. University of Washington. https://www.ncbi.nlm.nih.gov/books/NBK1252

FLCN (BIRT-HOGG-DUBÉ SYNDROME)

Cancer Risks

- For people with an *FLCN* pathogenic variant, risk of developing fibrofolliculomas is 84%, and most occur after age 20 years

- Risk of pulmonary cysts is approximately 85%, and most cysts probably start developing in childhood.
- Risk of a spontaneous pneumothorax is approximately 25%.
- Risk of renal cell cancer is 19%–35% and can include chromophobe, clear cell, hybrid oncocytic, and papillary types.
- Risk of malignant melanoma and thyroid, parotid, and colon cancer may be increased.

Management Options for Screening and Risk Reduction

Increased Screening

- Dermatologic examination every 6–12 months to monitor for malignant melanoma is recommended. Fibrofolliculomas generally do not require treatment.
- To decrease radiation exposure, routine screening for lung cysts is not indicated unless a patient has symptoms.
- A lung CT is indicated for those with suspected or previously treated pneumothorax, as well as prior to scheduled anesthesia or long-distance flights.
- Abdominal and pelvic MRI should start at age 20 years. This should be repeated annually in those with lesions smaller than 1 cm or complex cysts. For those without a history of renal cancer and three consecutive normal exams, the interval can increase to every two years. When a lesion reaches 3 cm, consideration can be given to nephron-sparing surgery.
- A physical examination should be performed to assess for parotid pain and thyroid masses. Annual thyroid ultrasound can be considered.
- Colonoscopy screening should start by age 40 years or 10 years prior to the age of the earliest cancer diagnosis in the family. Screening should be repeated every three to five years, depending on the number of polyps detected.

Risk-Reducing Surgery

- No recommendations

Other Preventive Measures

- Individuals should avoid tobacco use.
- Individuals should avoid high ambient pressures, especially air travel. High ambient pressures may precipitate spontaneous pneumothorax.
- Individuals should avoid radiation exposure.

Age to Test Relatives

- Approximately age 18 years

Reference

Sattler, E.C., & Steinlein, O.K. (2020). Birt-Hogg-Dubé syndrome. In M.P. Adam, H.H. Ardinger, R.A. Pagon, & S.E. Wallace (Eds.), *GeneReviews*®. University of Washington. https://www.ncbi.nlm.nih.gov/books/NBK1522

GREM1 AND *SCG5* (HEREDITARY MIXED POLYPOSIS SYNDROME)

Cancer Risks

- Individuals with a *GREM1* or *SCG5* pathogenic variant are at increased risk for developing colon cancer because of multiple polyps. Polyp types include juvenile-adenomatous colon polyps, adenomas, hyperplastic serrated adenomas, and mixed hyperplastic-adenomatous polyps.
- These pathogenic variants are much more common in people of Ashkenazi Jewish ancestry.

Management Options for Screening and Risk Reduction

Increased Screening

- Colonoscopy repeated every one to two years depending on whether polyps are detected, starting at age 25–30 years.

Risk-Reducing Surgery

- Consideration of colectomy if polyp burden becomes too high to manage with regular colonoscopy

Age to Test Relatives

- Approximately age 25 years

References

Jasperson, K.W., Patel, S.G., & Ahnen, D.J. (2017). *APC*-associated polyposis conditions. In M.P. Adam, H.H. Ardinger, R.A. Pagon, & S.E. Wallace (Eds.), *GeneReviews®*. University of Washington. https://www.ncbi.nlm.nih.gov/books/NBK1345

National Comprehensive Cancer Network. (2020). *NCCN Clinical Practice Guidelines in Oncology (NCCN Guidelines®): Genetic/familial high-risk assessment: Colorectal* [v.1.2020]. https://www.nccn.org/professionals/physician_gls/pdf/genetics_colon.pdf

HOXB13

Cancer Risks

- Men with an *HOXB13* pathogenic variant are at increased risk for developing prostate cancer.

Management Options for Screening and Risk Reduction

Increased Screening

- Early prostate screening with a rectal exam and a PSA blood test, starting by age 40 years

Risk-Reducing Surgery

- No recommendations

Age to Test Relatives

- Approximately age 25 years

References

Giri, V.N., Knudsen, K.E., Kelly, W.K., Abida, W., Andriole, G.L., Bangma, C.H., ... Gomella, L.G. (2018). Role of genetic testing for inherited prostate cancer risk: Philadelphia Prostate Cancer Consensus Conference 2017. *Journal of Clinical Oncology, 36*(4), 414–424. https://doi.org/10.1200/JCO.2017.74.1173

National Comprehensive Cancer Network. (2020). *NCCN Clinical Practice Guidelines in Oncology (NCCN Guidelines®): Prostate cancer early detection* [v.2.2020]. https://www.nccn.org/professionals/physician_gls/pdf/prostate_detection.pdf

MAX, SDHA, SDHAF2, SDHB, SDHC, SDHD, AND *TMEM127* (HEREDITARY PARAGANGLIOMA/PHEOCHROMOCYTOMA SYNDROME)

Cancer Risks

- *MAX* pathogenic variants are associated with the following risks:
  - Multiple pheochromocytomas are most commonly associated; 60% of those affected will have bilateral disease.
  - Occasionally, individuals develop paragangliomas but usually following a pheochromocytoma (25% risk of malignancy).
- *SDHA* pathogenic variants are associated with the following risks:
  - Pheochromocytomas and paragangliomas (both sympathetic and parasympathetic)
  - Risk of malignancy considered low
  - Gastrointestinal stromal tumors (GISTs) may occur.
- *SDHAF2* pathogenic variants are associated with the following risks:
  - Pathogenic variants have only been associated with head and neck paragangliomas; 90% of those affected will have more than one.
  - Risk of malignancy is unclear.

- *SDHB* pathogenic variants are associated with the following risks:
  - Pathogenic variants are associated with higher morbidity and mortality than pathogenic variants in the other *SDH* genes.
  - Pathogenic variants are strongly associated with extra-adrenal sympathetic paragangliomas, with an increased risk of metastatic disease and, less frequently, with pheochromocytomas and parasympathetic paragangliomas.
  - An estimated 20% of individuals with an *SDHB* pathogenic variant will have more than one paraganglioma.
  - Risk of tumors and malignancies in the kidneys is increased.
  - Overall risk of malignancy is estimated to be 37%–94%.
- *SDHC* pathogenic variants are associated with the following risks:
  - Pathogenic variants are primarily linked to head and neck paragangliomas, with approximately 10% of the paragangliomas in the thoracic cavity. An estimated 20% will have more than one paraganglioma, but risk of malignancy is estimated to be low.
  - GISTs may occur.
- *SDHD* pathogenic variants are associated with the following risks:
  - Pathogenic variants are primarily associated with head and neck paragangliomas, but extra-adrenal paragangliomas and pheochromocytomas can occur.
  - An estimated 50% will have more than one paraganglioma, but the risk of malignancy is less than 5%.
- *TMEM127* pathogenic variants are associated with the following risks:
  - Pathogenic variants are associated with adrenal pheochromocytomas; approximately 25% have bilateral disease. Pathogenic variants can also be linked to head and neck and extra-adrenal paraganglioma.
  - Renal cell carcinoma has also been reported.
  - Risk of malignancy is low.

Management Options for Screening and Risk Reduction

Increased Screening

- Annual measurement of plasma-free metanephrines and catecholamines to detect active catecholamine-secreting tumors or 24-hour urine collection for fractionated metanephrines
- Every two years, cross-sectional imaging of skull base to pelvis, ideally with MRI to reduce radiation exposure
- Endoscopy with esophagogastroduodenoscopy for evaluation for GISTs in patients with unexplained gastrointestinal symptoms (e.g., abdominal pain, upper gastrointestinal bleeding, nausea, vomiting, difficulty swallowing) or patients with unexplained intestinal obstruction or anemia

Risk-Reducing Surgery

- No recommendations

Other Preventive Measures

- Patient education about the following symptoms, which should be reported and evaluated promptly:
  - Gastrointestinal bleeding, difficulty swallowing, and unexplained nausea or vomiting
  - High or variable blood pressure, especially spiking blood pressure
  - Increase in frequency or intensity of headaches
  - Increased sweating or what feels like a panic attack, fear, or anxiety
  - Irregular or rapid heartbeat
  - Loss of balance or coordination
  - Loss of bowel or bladder function
  - Loss of hearing
  - Pain, including abdominal pain, of unknown cause

Age to Test Relatives

- Approximately age 5–10 years

References

Else, T., Greenberg, S., & Fishbein, L. (2018). Hereditary paraganglioma-pheochromocytoma syndromes. In M.P. Adam, H.H. Ardinger, R.A. Pagon, & S.E. Wallace (Eds.), *GeneReviews®*. University of Washington. https://www.ncbi.nlm.nih.gov/books/NBK1548

Lenders, J.W.M., Duh, Q.-Y., Eisenhofer, G., Gimenez-Roqueplo, A.-P., Grebe, S.K.G., Murad, M.H., ... Young, W.F., Jr. (2014). Pheochromocytoma and paraganglioma: An Endocrine Society clinical practice guideline. *Journal of Clinical Endocrinology and Metabolism, 99*(6), 1915–1942. https://doi.org/10.1210/jc.2014-1498

MEN1 (MULTIPLE ENDOCRINE NEOPLASIA TYPE 1)

Cancer Risks

- Individuals with a *MEN1* pathogenic variant are at increased risk for developing parathyroid tumors (lifetime risk of 88%–97%), with most having primary hypercalcemia and primary hyperparathyroidism by age 50 years.
- People with a pathogenic variant are at increased risk for pituitary tumors (lifetime risk of 30%–84%), with prolactinoma manifesting as oligomenorrhea, amenorrhea, or galactorrhea in females and sexual dysfunction in males.
- Individuals are at increased risk for gastroenteropancreatic gastrinoma (lifetime risk of 40%), which can manifest as the following:
  - Hyperglycemia, anorexia, glossitis, anemia, diarrhea, venous thrombosis, and skin rash (glucagonoma)
  - Hypoglycemia (insulinoma)
  - Watery diarrhea, hypokalemia, and achlorhydria syndrome (vasoactive intestinal peptide–secreting tumor)
  - Zollinger-Ellison syndrome (gastrinoma)

- Those with a pathogenic variant are at increased risk for facial angiofibromas, collagenomas, lipomas, ependymomas, meningiomas, and leiomyomas.

Management Options for Screening and Risk Reduction

Increased Screening

- Serum prolactin, starting at age five years
- MRI of the head, starting at age five years
- Serum glucose, insulin, and proinsulin, starting at age five years
- Serum concentrations of calcium, starting at age eight years
- Serum parathyroid hormone, starting at age eight years
- Monitoring of fasting and meal-stimulated pancreatic polypeptide, starting at age eight years
- Abdominal and chest CT or MRI every two to three years starting at age 20 years
- Fasting serum gastrin, starting at age 20 years. If gastrin is elevated, a secretin-stimulated gastrin test is indicated.

Risk-Reducing Surgery

- Parathyroidectomy is the treatment of choice for individuals with a *MEN1* pathogenic variant, but it is controversial whether to perform subtotal (less than 3.5 glands) or total parathyroidectomy and whether surgery should be performed at an early or late stage of the disease.
- Thymectomy may prevent thymic carcinoid in men and can be considered at the time of parathyroid neck surgery, particularly in smokers and individuals with a family history of thymic carcinoma.

Age to Test Relatives

- Approximately age three years

References

Giusti, F., Marini, F., & Brandi, M.L. (2017). Multiple endocrine neoplasia type 1. In M.P. Adam, H.H. Ardinger, R.A. Pagon, & S.E. Wallace (Eds.), *GeneReviews®*. University of Washington. https://www.ncbi.nlm.nih.gov/books/NBK1538

National Comprehensive Cancer Network. (2020). *NCCN Clinical Practice Guidelines in Oncology (NCCN Guidelines®): Neuroendocrine and adrenal tumors* [v.2.2020]. https://www.nccn.org/professionals/physician_gls/pdf/neuroendocrine.pdf

MEN2 (MULTIPLE ENDOCRINE NEOPLASIA TYPE 2)

Cancer Risks

- Three subtypes of *MEN2* pathogenic variants are commonly associated with cancer risk:

- *MEN2* familial medullary thyroid carcinoma has a 100% risk of developing cancer.
- *MEN2A* is associated with a 95%–100% risk of medullary thyroid cancer, a 40%–50% risk of pheochromocytoma, a 10%–30% risk of primary hyperparathyroidism, an increased risk of Hirschsprung disease, and an increased risk of cutaneous lichen amyloidosis
- *MEN2B* is associated with a 100% risk of medullary thyroid cancer; a 100% risk of mucosal-intestinal ganglioneuromas; a 100% risk of Marfanoid habitus; a 100% risk of mucosal neuromas in the tongue, lips, and eyelids; and a 50% risk of pheochromocytoma.

Management Options for Screening and Risk Reduction

Increased Screening

- Annual measurement of serum calcitonin, even following thyroidectomy
- Beginning at age eight years, annual 24-hour urine collection to measure levels of catecholamines and metanephrines, as well as neck ultrasound
- Consideration of annual chest and abdominal CT or MRI
- Annual biochemical screening for parathyroid adenoma, starting by age eight years, including serum calcium, parathyroid hormone, 25-hydroxyvitamin D_3, calcitonin, and metanephrines.

Risk-Reducing Surgery

- Prophylactic thyroidectomy between six months and five years of age for individuals with a germline *MEN2* pathogenic variant

Other Preventive Measures

- Individuals should avoid dopamine D_2 receptor antagonists and beta-blockers. These drugs are associated with a high risk for adverse reactions in individuals with pheochromocytoma.
- Individuals should be educated about the following symptoms, which should be reported and evaluated promptly:
  - High or variable blood pressure, especially spiking blood pressure
  - Increase in frequency or intensity of headaches
  - Increased sweating or what feels like a panic attack, fear, or anxiety
  - Irregular or rapid heartbeat

Age to Test Relatives

- By age one year

References

Eng, C. (2019). Multiple endocrine neoplasia type 2. In M.P. Adam, H.H. Ardinger, R.A. Pagon, & S.E. Wallace (Eds.), *GeneReviews®*. University of Washington. https://www.ncbi.nlm.nih.gov/books/NBK1257

National Comprehensive Cancer Network. (2020). *NCCN Clinical Practice Guidelines in Oncology (NCCN Guidelines®): Neuroendocrine and adrenal tumors* [v.2.2020]. https://www.nccn.org/professionals/physician_gls/pdf/neuroendocrine.pdf
Wells, S.A., Jr., Asa, S.L., Dralle, H., Elisei, R., Evans, D.B., Gagel, R.F., ... Waguespack, S.G. (2015). Revised American Thyroid Association guidelines for the management of medullary thyroid carcinoma. *Thyroid, 25*(6), 567–610. https://doi.org/10.1089/thy.2014.0335

MET

Cancer Risks

- Risk of papillary renal cell cancer approaches 100% for people with a pathogenic variant of *MET*.
- Individuals have an increased risk of nonsyndromic hearing loss.
- *MET* variance may be associated with hepatocellular carcinoma, lung cancer, and the development of a highly malignant, metastatic syndrome known as cancer of unknown primary origin or primary occult malignancy.

Management Options for Screening and Risk Reduction

Increased Screening
- If kidney function is normal and a patient has no allergy to contrast, cross-sectional imaging with CT or MRI is the best initial imaging technique for identifying hypovascular renal tumors, which are often missed with renal ultrasonography.
- MRI of the kidneys is typically recommended as an imaging modality to minimize the lifetime dose of radiation and can be performed every three to five years. If a tumor smaller than 3 cm is found, imaging should be repeated within the first year to assess the growth rate. Based on growth characteristics and tumor size, imaging frequency can be adapted to prevent the largest tumor from exceeding 3 cm. When the tumor reaches 3 cm in size, surgery should be considered.

Risk-Reducing Surgery
- No recommendations

Other Preventive Measures
- Individuals should avoid tobacco use, as it is estimated to double the risk of papillary renal cancer.

Age to Test Relatives
- Approximately age 25 years

References

Haas, N.B., & Nathanson, K.L. (2014). Hereditary kidney cancer syndromes. *Advances in Chronic Kidney Disease, 21*(1), 81–90. https://doi.org/10.1053/j.ackd.2013.10.001

National Cancer Institute. (2020). Genetics of kidney cancer (renal cell cancer) (PDQ®) [Health professional version]. https://www.cancer.gov/types/kidney/hp/kidney-genetics-pdq

U.S. National Library of Medicine. (2020). MET—MET proto-oncogene, receptor tyrosine kinase. In *Gene*. https://www.ncbi.nlm.nih.gov/gene/4233

MITF

Cancer Risks

- Individuals with a *MITF* pathogenic variant are at increased risk for developing melanoma.

Management Options for Screening and Risk Reduction

Increased Screening

- Full body skin examination for melanoma screening, with frequency (annual at minimum) depending on personal and family history of melanoma and atypical moles. Whole-body skin photography may be helpful in individuals with many moles.
- Monthly self-examination of the skin

Risk-Reducing Surgery

- None

Other Preventive Measures

- Individuals should avoid artificial tanning.
- When in the sun, individuals should avoid sunburns by using broad-spectrum (UVA/UVB) sunscreen of SPF of 30 or higher, seeking shade, covering up with clothing (including hats), and wearing UV-blocking sunglasses.

Age to Test Relatives

- Approximately age 25 years

References

Read, J., Wadt, K.A.W., & Hayward, N.K. (2016). Melanoma genetics. *Journal of Medical Genetics, 53*(1), 1–14. https://doi.org/10.1136/jmedgenet-2015-103150

U.S. National Library of Medicine. (2020). MITF gene. In *MedlinePlus*. https://ghr.nlm.nih.gov/gene/MITF

MUTYH

Cancer Risks

- Individuals with homozygous (two altered copies of the gene) pathogenic variants of *MUTYH* have the following risks:
  - Bladder cancer risk is 6%–8% in women and 6%–25% in men, with a mean age at diagnosis of 61 years.
  - Breast cancer risk is 12%–25% in women, with a mean age at diagnosis of 53 years.
  - Colon cancer risk is estimated to be 43%–63% by age 60 years. Lifetime risk of colon cancer is 80%–90%, with a mean age at diagnosis of 48 years.
  - Duodenal cancer risk is 4%, with a mean age at diagnosis of 61 years.
  - Endometrial cancer risk is approximately 3%, with a mean age at diagnosis of 51 years.
  - Ovarian cancer risk is 6%–14%, with a mean age at diagnosis of 51 years.
  - Risk of gastric cancer is approximately 1%, with a mean age at diagnosis of 38 years.
  - Risk of skin (melanoma and nonmelanoma), thyroid, and pancreatic cancer may be increased.
- Individuals with a heterozygous (one altered and one working copy of the gene) pathogenic variant of *MUTYH* have the following risks:
  - Colon cancer risk is increased.
  - Gastric, hepatobiliary, endometrial, and breast cancer risk may be increased.

Management Options for Screening and Risk Reduction

Increased Screening

- Colonoscopy with polypectomy, starting at approximately age 25 years
  - For homozygotes, screening should occur every one to two years, depending on polyp burden.
  - For heterozygotes, screening should occur every three to five years depending on polyp burden.
- Upper endoscopy and side viewing duodenoscopy every three months to four years starting by age 30 years, depending on polyp burden
  - For homozygotes, the stomach should be visualized at the time of upper endoscopy.
  - For heterozygotes, there is no specific recommendation, but it can be performed at the time of colonoscopy.
- Annual physical examination, including evaluation for extraintestinal manifestations, including a full body skin examination and palpation of thyroid
- Mammography, starting by age 40 years or 10 years before the age of earliest diagnosis of breast cancer in the family
- Annual breast examination and prompt evaluation of any change

- Annual gynecologic examination with consideration of pelvic ultrasound to evaluate the ovaries and endometrium

Risk-Reducing Surgery

- There is an absolute indication for colectomy when colorectal cancer is diagnosed or suspected or when significant symptoms (e.g., bleeding, obstruction) occur.
- Relative indications for colectomy include the following:
  - Presence of multiple adenomas larger than 6 mm that cannot be reasonably removed endoscopically
  - Significant increase in adenoma number between surveillance exams
  - Presence of adenomas with high-grade dysplasia
  - Inability to adequately survey the colon (e.g., due to innumerous diminutive adenomas, limited access to or compliance with colonoscopy)

Other Preventive Measures

- Colonoscopy is used for surveillance and prevention of colon cancer.
- To reduce the risk of duodenal and periampullary adenocarcinoma, endoscopic or surgical removal of duodenal and ampullary adenomas should be considered if polyps exhibit villous change or severe dysplasia, exceed 1 cm in diameter, or cause symptoms.
- Individuals should avoid tobacco use, which is associated with an increased risk for developing colon and bladder cancers

Age to Test Relatives

- Approximately age 25 years

References

National Comprehensive Cancer Network. (2020). *NCCN Clinical Practice Guidelines in Oncology (NCCN Guidelines®): Genetic/familial high-risk assessment: Colorectal* [v.1.2020]. https://www.nccn.org/professionals/physician_gls/pdf/genetics_colon.pdf

Nielsen, M., Infante, E., & Brand, R. (2019). *MUTYH* polyposis. In M.P. Adam, H.H. Ardinger, R.A. Pagon, & S.E. Wallace (Eds.), *GeneReviews®*. University of Washington. https://www.ncbi.nlm.nih.gov/books/NBK107219

NBN, MRE11A, AND *RAD50*

Cancer Risks

- Individuals with homozygous pathogenic variants of *NBN*, *MRE11A*, or *RAD50* have the following risks:
  - Homozygotes have a condition known as Nijmegen breakage syndrome, which is characterized by progressive microcephaly, intrauterine growth retardation

and short stature, recurrent sinopulmonary infections, and premature ovarian failure in females. Intellectual abilities tend to decline over time, and by age seven years, most children have mild to moderate intellectual disability. Recurrent pneumonia and bronchitis may result in respiratory failure and early death.
  - Approximately 40% of individuals with Nijmegen breakage syndrome develop malignancies before age 20 years, with the risk being highest for T-cell lymphomas (55%) and B-cell lymphomas (45%). The lifetime risk of developing ovarian cancer is increased.
- Individuals with heterozygous pathogenic variants of *NBN*, *MRE11A*, or *RAD50* have the following risks:
  - For men, the risk of developing prostate cancer is increased.
  - For women, the risk of developing breast cancer is increased.
  - For women, the risk of developing ovarian cancer may be increased.

Management Options for Screening and Risk Reduction

Increased Screening

- Mammography and breast MRI, alternating every six months, starting by age 30 years
- Clinical breast exam (ideally by a breast surgeon) every 6–12 months, starting at age 25 years
- Monthly breast self-examination starting at age 18 years, with prompt evaluation of any change
- Early prostate screening with a rectal exam of the prostate and a PSA blood test, starting at age 40, especially in men with an *NBN* pathogenic variant and those with a family history of prostate cancer

Risk-Reducing Surgery

- Bilateral risk-reducing mastectomy with an option for breast reconstruction. Surgery reduces the chance of developing breast cancer by at least 95% and is typically reserved for families with an extensive history of early-onset breast cancer and those diagnosed with breast cancer.

Other Preventive Measures

- Preconception testing is recommended for heterozygotes to clarify risk of having a child with Nijmegen breakage syndrome.

Age to Test Other Relatives

- Approximately age 25 years

References

National Comprehensive Cancer Network. (2020). *NCCN Clinical Practice Guidelines in Oncology (NCCN Guidelines®): Genetic/familial high-risk assessment: Breast, ovarian, and pancreatic* [v.2.2021]. https://www.nccn.org/professionals/physician_gls/pdf/genetics_bop.pdf

Varon, R., Demuth, I., & Chrzanowska, K.H. (2017). Nijmegen breakage syndrome. In M.P. Adam, H.H. Ardinger, R.A. Pagon, & S.E. Wallace (Eds.), *GeneReviews®*. University of Washington. https://www.ncbi.nlm.nih.gov/books/NBK1176

NTHL1

Cancer Risks

- Individuals with a homozygous pathogenic variant of *NTHL1* have the following risks:
  - Risk of breast cancer is increased.
  - Risk of cervical cancer, urothelial carcinoma of the bladder, meningiomas, brain tumors, basal cell carcinomas, head and neck squamous cell carcinomas, and hematologic cancers is increased.
  - Risk of colon polyps and colon cancer is increased. Mean age at diagnosis of colon cancer is approximately 60 years, with a range of 30–75 years.
  - Risk of duodenal polyps and cancers may be increased.
  - Risk of endometrial cancer is increased.
  - Risk of skin hemangiomas, seborrheic keratosis, intradermal nevi, ovarian and hepatic cysts, and breast papillomas may be increased.
- Individuals with a heterozygous pathogenic variant of *NTHL1* have an increased risk of colon cancer.

Management Options for Screening and Risk Reduction

Increased Screening

- Colonoscopy with polypectomy, starting at age 18 years
  - For homozygotes, screening should occur every two years, depending on polyp burden.
  - For heterozygotes, screening should occur every three to five years, depending on polyp burden.
- Upper endoscopy and side-viewing duodenoscopy, starting by age 25 years, depending on polyp burden
  - For homozygotes, the stomach should be visualized at the time of upper endoscopy.
  - For heterozygotes, there is no specific recommendation, but upper endoscopy can be done at the time of colonoscopy.
- Annual physical examination, including evaluation for extraintestinal manifestations, including a total body skin examination and neurologic examination
- Annual mammography, starting at age 40 years or 10 years prior to the age of the youngest breast cancer diagnosis in the family
- Annual breast examination and prompt evaluation of any change

- In homozygotes, consideration of alternating breast MRI with mammography every six months
- Annual gynecologic examination, with consideration for pelvic ultrasound to evaluate the ovaries and endometrium

Risk-Reducing Surgery

- There is an absolute indication for colectomy when colorectal cancer is diagnosed or suspected or when significant symptoms (e.g., bleeding, obstruction) are present.
- Relative indications for colectomy include the following:
  - Presence of multiple adenomas larger than 6 mm that cannot be reasonably removed endoscopically
  - Significant increase in adenomas between surveillance exams
  - Presence of adenomas with high-grade dysplasia
  - Inability to adequately survey the colon (e.g., due to innumerous diminutive adenomas, limited access to or compliance with colonoscopy)

Other Preventive Measures

- Colonoscopy is used for surveillance and prevention of colon cancer.
- To reduce the risk of duodenal and periampullary adenocarcinoma, endoscopic or surgical removal of duodenal and ampullary adenomas should be considered if polyps exhibit villous change or severe dysplasia, exceed 1 cm in diameter, or cause symptoms.
- Individuals should avoid tobacco use, which is associated with an increased risk for developing colon and bladder cancers.

Age to Test Relatives

- Approximately age 18 years

References

Kuiper, R.P., Nielsen, M., De Over, R.M., & Hoogerbrugge, N. (2020). *NTHL1* tumor syndrome. In M.P. Adam, H.H. Ardinger, R.A. Pagon, & S.E. Wallace (Eds.), *GeneReviews®*. University of Washington. https://www.ncbi.nlm.nih.gov/books/NBK555473

National Comprehensive Cancer Network. (2020). *NCCN Clinical Practice Guidelines in Oncology (NCCN Guidelines®): Genetic/familial high-risk assessment: Colorectal* [v.1.2020]. https://www.nccn.org/professionals/physician_gls/pdf/genetics_colon.pdf

NF1 (NEUROFIBROMATOSIS TYPE 1)

Cancer Risks

- Neurofibromatosis type 1 should be suspected in individuals who have two or more of the following findings:

- Six or more café-au-lait macules larger than 5 mm in greatest diameter in prepubertal individuals and greater than 15 mm in greatest diameter in postpubertal individuals
- Freckling in the axillary or inguinal region
- Optic glioma
- Two or more Lisch nodules (iris hamartomas)
- Distinctive osseous lesion, such as sphenoid dysplasia or tibial pseudoarthrosis
- First-degree relative with neurofibromatosis type 1

• Risk of a malignant nerve sheath tumor or GIST may be as high as 60%.
• Women have increased risk for developing breast cancer, especially before the age of 50 years.

Management Options for Screening and Risk Reduction

Increased Screening

• Annual physical examination by a physician who is familiar with neurofibromatosis type 1
• Annual ophthalmologic examination, starting in early childhood
• Regular developmental assessment by screening questionnaire and observation in children
• Regular blood pressure monitoring, starting at age five years
• Monitoring by an appropriate specialist of individuals with abnormalities of the central nervous system, skeletal system, or cardiovascular system
• Annual mammography, starting at age 30 years
• Consideration of breast MRI during age 30–50 years, alternating every six months with mammography
• Clinical breast exam (ideally by a breast surgeon) every 6–12 months, starting at age 25 years
• Monthly breast self-examination starting at age 18 years, with prompt evaluation of any change

Risk-Reducing Surgery

• Consideration of risk-reducing mastectomies in people with a significant family history

Other Preventive Measures

• Precautions should be taken if a patient receives radiation therapy because it is associated with a high risk of developing malignant peripheral nerve sheath tumors within the treatment field.

Age to Test Relatives

• Diagnosis is often made by clinical symptoms.
• Testing can be performed around age five years.

References

Friedman, J.M. (2019). Neurofibromatosis 1. In M.P. Adam, H.H. Ardinger, R.A. Pagon, & S.E. Wallace (Eds.), *GeneReviews®*. University of Washington. https://www.ncbi.nlm.nih.gov/books/NBK1109

National Comprehensive Cancer Network. (2020). *NCCN Clinical Practice Guidelines in Oncology (NCCN Guidelines®): Genetic/familial high-risk assessment: Breast, ovarian, and pancreatic* [v.2.2021]. https://www.nccn.org/professionals/physician_gls/pdf/genetics_bop.pdf

NF2 (NEUROFIBROMATOSIS TYPE 2)

Cancer Risks

- Individuals with neurofibromatosis type 2 have an increased risk of bilateral vestibular schwannomas, which result in tinnitus, hearing loss, and balance dysfunction. These occur in nearly all affected individuals by age 30 years, with the average age at onset being 18–24 years.
- Affected individuals are at increased risk for developing schwannomas of other cranial and peripheral nerves, meningiomas, ependymomas, and, very rarely, astrocytomas.

Management Options for Screening and Risk Reduction

Increased Screening

- Annual cranial MRI, starting at age 10–12 years and continuing until at least the fourth decade of life
- Annual hearing evaluation, including brain stem auditory evoked response testing. Screening may be useful in detecting changes in auditory nerve function before changes can be visualized by MRI.
- Annual complete eye examination for all individuals with neurofibromatosis type 2
- Annual physical examination, ideally by a specialist familiar with neurofibromatosis type 2

Risk-Reducing Surgery

- No recommendations

Other Preventive Measures

- Precautions should be taken if a patient receives radiation therapy because it is associated with an increased risk of developing malignant tumors, especially within the treatment field.

Age to Test Relatives

- Age 5–10 years

Reference

Evans, D.G. (2018). Neurofibromatosis 2. In M.P. Adam, H.H. Ardinger, R.A. Pagon, & S.E. Wallace (Eds.), *GeneReviews®*. University of Washington. https://www.ncbi.nlm.nih.gov/books/NBK1201

PALB2

Cancer Risks

- Women with a *PALB2* pathogenic variant have a 58% chance of developing breast cancer, compared to 12% in the general population.
- Men with a *PALB2* pathogenic variant are at increased risk for developing breast cancer.
- For women, risk of ovarian cancer may be increased.
- For men and women, risk of pancreatic cancer is increased.

Management Options for Screening and Risk Reduction

Increased Screening

- Annual mammography starting by age 30 years, with consideration of breast MRI alternating every six months with mammography
- Clinical breast exam (ideally by a breast surgeon) every 6–12 months, starting at age 25 years
- Monthly breast self-examination starting at age 18 years, with prompt evaluation of any change
- Transvaginal ultrasound screening of the ovaries and a CA-125 blood test every six months, starting at approximately age 30 years
- In men, annual clinical breast exam by a healthcare provider, beginning at age 25 years
- In men, monthly breast self-examination starting at age 35 years
- In men and women, annual pancreatic screening starting at age 40 years or 10 years prior to the age of the earliest pancreatic cancer diagnosis in the family, with MRI/MRCP, EUS, fasting blood glucose, and HbA1c. Annual recommended follow-up includes alternating MRI/MRCP and EUS with annual fasting blood glucose and HbA1c.

Risk-Reducing Surgery

- Bilateral risk-reducing mastectomy with an option of breast reconstruction for women with a family history of breast cancer
- Consideration of surgery to remove the ovaries and fallopian tubes at age 40–45 years, when childbearing is complete, especially for women with a family history of ovarian cancer

Other Preventive Measures

- Tamoxifen and raloxifene, medications used to treat breast cancer, have been shown to reduce the risk of certain types of breast cancer by up to 50%. Individuals can consider using these medications for five years.

Age to Test Relatives

- Approximately age 25 years

References

Goggins, M., Overbeek, K.A., Brand, R., Syngal, S., Del Chiaro, M., Bartsch, D.K., ... Bruno, M. (2020). Management of patients with increased risk for familial pancreatic cancer: Updated recommendations from the International Cancer of the Pancreas Screening (CAPS) Consortium. *Gut, 69*(1), 7–17. https://doi.org/10.1136/gutjnl-2019-319352

National Comprehensive Cancer Network. (2020). *NCCN Clinical Practice Guidelines in Oncology (NCCN Guidelines®): Genetic/familial high-risk assessment: Breast, ovarian, and pancreatic* [v.2.2021]. https://www.nccn.org/professionals/physician_gls/pdf/genetics_bop.pdf

Petrucelli, N., Daly, M.B., & Pal, T. (2016). *BRCA1*- and *BRCA2*-associated hereditary breast and ovarian cancer. In M.P. Adam, H.H. Ardinger, R.A. Pagon, & S.E. Wallace (Eds.), *GeneReviews®*. University of Washington. https://www.ncbi.nlm.nih.gov/books/NBK1247

POLD1 AND *POLE1*

Cancer Risks

- *POLD1* and *POLE1* pathogenic variants are associated with an increased risk of colon polyps. Cases of early onset (before age 45 years) have been reported, but the exact risk is unknown.
- Risk for breast and endometrial cancer may be increased with *POLD1* pathogenic variants.

Management Options for Screening and Risk Reduction

Increased Screening

- Colonoscopy every one to three years, depending on whether polyps are detected, starting at age 25–30 years
- Annual clinical breast exam, starting at age 25 years
- Monthly breast self-examination starting at age 18 years, with prompt evaluation of any change
- Annual mammography, starting by age 40 years (earlier for a family history of breast cancer)
- Careful gynecologic examination annually and prompt evaluation of any unexplained spotting, bleeding, or discharge

Risk-Reducing Surgery

- Relative indications for colectomy include the following:
  - Presence of multiple adenomas larger than 6 mm that cannot be reasonably removed endoscopically
  - Significant increase in adenomas between surveillance exams
  - Presence of adenomas with high-grade dysplasia
  - Inability to adequately survey the colon (e.g., due to innumerous diminutive adenomas, limited access to or compliance with colonoscopy)

Age to Test Relatives

- Approximately age 20–25 years

Reference

National Comprehensive Cancer Network. (2020). *NCCN Clinical Practice Guidelines in Oncology (NCCN Guidelines®): Genetic/familial high-risk assessment: Colorectal* [v.1.2020]. https://www.nccn.org/professionals/physician_gls/pdf/genetics_colon.pdf

POT1

Cancer Risks

- *POT1* pathogenic variants are associated with an increased risk of developing early-onset melanoma.
- There may be an increased risk of benign and malignant gliomas.

Management Options for Screening and Risk Reduction

Increased Screening

- Full body skin examination for melanoma screening with the frequency (at least annually) depending on personal and family history of melanoma and atypical moles. Whole-body skin photography may be helpful in individuals with many moles.
- Monthly self-examination of the skin

Risk-Reducing Surgery

- No recommendations

Other Preventive Measures

- Individuals should avoid artificial tanning.

- When in the sun, individuals should avoid sunburns by using broad-spectrum (UVA/UVB) sunscreen of SPF 30 or higher, seeking shade, covering up with clothing (including hats), and wearing UV-blocking sunglasses.

Age to Test Relatives
- Approximately age 25 years

References

Read, J., Wadt, K.A.W., & Hayward, N.K. (2016). Melanoma genetics. *Journal of Medical Genetics, 53*(1), 1–14. https://doi.org/10.1136/jmedgenet-2015-103150

U.S. National Library of Medicine. (2020). POT1—Protection of telomeres 1. In *Gene*. https://www.ncbi.nlm.nih.gov/gene/25913

PTCH1 AND *SUFU* (NEVOID BASAL CELL CARCINOMA SYNDROME)

Cancer Risks

- Individuals with a *PTCH1* pathogenic variant have the following risks:
  - Risk of basal cell cancer is 100%, with many being very early onset.
  - Individuals typically have jaw cysts (90% with multiple cysts) and bifid ribs.
  - An estimated 60% of individuals have a distinct appearance with frontal bossing, coarse facial features, and facial milia.
  - Risk of medulloblastoma is approximately 2%.
- Individuals with an *SUFU* pathogenic variant have the following risks:
  - Risk for basal cell cancer is high but typically less than with *PTCH1* pathogenic variants.
  - Risk for medulloblastoma is approximately 33%.
  - Facial features are likely more subtle in individuals with an *SUFU* pathogenic variant, and jaw cysts are not seen.

Management Options for Screening and Risk Reduction

Increased Screening
- Baseline measurement of head circumference, preferably plotted on a chart that accounts for height. Evidence of rapid increase in centiles should prompt further investigation to exclude hydrocephalus.
- Physical examination for birth defects of clinical significance (e.g., orofacial clefts, polydactyly)

- X-rays to evaluate for rib and vertebral anomalies and falx calcification
- Ophthalmologic evaluation for evidence of strabismus, cataract, orbital cyst, microphthalmia, and pigmentary changes of the retinal epithelium
- Evaluation by a dentist or orthodontist with jaw x-ray (orthopantomogram) in individuals age eight years and older to evaluate for jaw keratocysts and other anomalies
- Skin examination by a dermatologist familiar with nevoid basal cell cardinoma syndrome, at least every six months
- Echocardiography in the first year of life to evaluate for cardiac fibromas

Risk-Reducing Surgery
- No recommendations

Other Preventive Measures
- Individuals should avoid artificial tanning.
- When in the sun, individuals should avoid sunburns by using broad-spectrum (UVA/UVB) sunscreen of SPF 30 or higher, seeking shade, covering up with clothing (including hats), and wearing UV-blocking sunglasses.
- Individuals should avoid radiation exposure.

Age to Test Relatives
- At birth

Reference

Evans, D.G., & Farndon, P.A. (2018). Nevoid basal cell carcinoma syndrome. In M.P. Adam, H.H. Ardinger, R.A. Pagon, & S.E. Wallace (Eds.), *GeneReviews®*. University of Washington. https://www.ncbi.nlm.nih.gov/books/NBK1151

PTEN (COWDEN SYNDROME)

Cancer Risks

- Women with a *PTEN* pathogenic variant have a 25%–80% chance of developing breast cancer. Mean age at diagnosis is 38–50 years.
- Risk of benign thyroid nodules is 30%–68%, and risk of thyroid cancer is 13%–28%.
- The lifetime risk of developing endometrial cancer is 5%–19%.
- Risk of kidney cancer is estimated to be 15%–34%.
- For men and women, the lifetime risk of colon cancer is 13%–16%.
- Risk of melanoma is 6%.

Management Options for Screening and Risk Reduction

Increased Screening

- Annual breast MRI (or mammography if MRI is unavailable) starting at age 25–29 years. At age 30 years and beyond, annual mammography and breast MRI are recommended, alternating every six months.
- Clinical breast exam (ideally by a breast surgeon) every 6–12 months, starting at age 25 years
- Monthly breast self-examination starting at age 18 years, with prompt evaluation of any change
- Transvaginal ultrasound screening of the endometrium and endometrial biopsy starting at age 35 years
- Annual thyroid examination, starting at age seven years
- Colonoscopy, starting by age 30 or 10 years prior to the age of the earliest colon cancer diagnosis in the family. It should be repeated every three to five years or more frequently depending on the polyp burden.
- Consideration of renal ultrasound every one to two years, starting by age 40 years
- Full body skin examination for melanoma screening, with frequency depending on personal and family history of melanoma and atypical moles
- Monthly self-examination of the skin

Risk-Reducing Surgery

- Bilateral risk-reducing mastectomy with an option of breast reconstruction. Surgery reduces the chance of developing breast cancer by at least 95%.
- Surgery to remove the uterus at age 35–45 years, when childbearing is complete

Other Preventive Measures

- Tamoxifen and raloxifene, medications used to treat breast cancer, have been shown to reduce the risk of certain types of breast cancer by up to 50%. Individuals can consider using these drugs for five years.
- Individuals should avoid artificial tanning.
- When in the sun, individuals should avoid sunburns by using broad-spectrum (UVA/UVB) sunscreen of SPF 30 or higher, seeking shade, covering up with clothing (including hats), and wearing UV-blocking sunglasses.

Age to Test Relatives

- Approximately age five years

References

Eng, C. (2016). *PTEN* hamartoma tumor syndrome. In M.P. Adam, H.H. Ardinger, R.A. Pagon, & S.E. Wallace (Eds.), *GeneReviews®*. University of Washington. https://www.ncbi.nlm.nih.gov/books/NBK1488

National Comprehensive Cancer Network. (2020). *NCCN Clinical Practice Guidelines in Oncology (NCCN Guidelines®): Genetic/familial high-risk assessment: Breast, ovarian, and pancreatic* [v.2.2021]. https://www.nccn.org/professionals/physician_gls/pdf/genetics_bop.pdf

RAD51C AND *RAD51D*

Cancer Risks

- Women with a *RAD51C* or *RAD51D* pathogenic variant have a potentially increased risk of breast cancer, especially triple-negative breast cancer.
- Risk of ovarian cancer is increased.

Management Options for Screening and Risk Reduction

Increased Screening

- Annual mammography and breast MRI, alternating every six months starting at age 30 years
- Clinical breast exam (ideally by a breast surgeon) every 6–12 months starting at age 25 years
- Monthly breast self-examination starting at age 18 years, with prompt evaluation of any change
- Transvaginal ultrasound screening of the ovaries and a CA-125 blood test every 6–12 months starting at approximately age 30 years, especially in those with a family history of ovarian cancer

Risk-Reducing Surgery

- Bilateral risk-reducing mastectomy with an option of breast reconstruction for women with a significant family history of breast cancer
- Surgery to remove the ovaries and fallopian tubes at age 40–45 years, when childbearing is complete, especially in those with a family history of ovarian cancer

Age to Test Relatives

- Approximately age 25 years

Reference

National Comprehensive Cancer Network. (2020). *NCCN Clinical Practice Guidelines in Oncology (NCCN Guidelines®): Genetic/familial high-risk assessment: Breast, ovarian, and pancreatic* [v.2.2021]. https://www.nccn.org/professionals/physician_gls/pdf/genetics_bop.pdf

RB1

Cancer Risks

- Approximately 60% of individuals affected with an *RB1* pathogenic variant have unilateral retinoblastoma, with a mean age at diagnosis of 24 months.
- Approximately 40% of individuals with an *RB1* pathogenic variant have bilateral retinoblastoma, with a mean age at diagnosis of 15 months.
- Risk of osteosarcomas and soft tissue sarcomas (mostly leiomyosarcomas and rhabdomyosarcomas) is increased.
- Risk of melanomas may also be increased.

Management Options for Screening and Risk Reduction

Increased Screening

- It is recommended that children who are known to have an *RB1* germline pathogenic variant have an eye examination under anesthesia every three to four weeks until age six months, then less frequently until age three years. Clinical examinations with cooperative children are performed every three to six months until age seven years, then annually for life.
- Because of the high risk of second cancers, including sarcomas and other uncommon cancers, prompt investigation of any signs or symptoms is indicated. Total-body MRI at regular intervals is under investigation to determine when the technology will be specific and sensitive enough for screening for second cancers in people with an *RB1* pathogenic variant.
- An annual dermatologic examination is recommended.

Risk-Reducing Surgery

- No recommendations

Other Preventive Measures

- If possible, any radiation (including x-ray, CT scan, and external beam radiation) should be avoided to minimize the lifetime risk of developing late-onset second cancers. Such tests should only be used if absolutely necessary in health care.
- Individuals should avoid artificial tanning.
- When out in the sun, individuals should avoid sunburns by using broad-spectrum (UVA/UVB) sunscreen of SPF 30 or higher, seeking shade, covering up with clothing (including hats), and wearing UV-blocking sunglasses.

Age to Test Relatives

- Testing should occur as soon as possible after birth, with an ocular exam to be performed while waiting for results.

- For families with a known *RB1* pathogenic variant, prenatal testing is possible. If an *RB1* pathogenic variant is identified in the fetus, ultrasound examination may be used to identify medium-sized intraocular tumors. If tumors are present, preterm delivery to enable early treatment may be considered.

Reference

Lohmann, D.R., & Gallie, B.L. (2018). Retinoblastoma. In M.P. Adam, H.H. Ardinger, R.A. Pagon, & S.E. Wallace (Eds.), *GeneReviews®*. University of Washington. https://www.ncbi.nlm.nih.gov/books/NBK1452

RECQL

Cancer Risks

- Women with an *RECQL* pathogenic variant may have an increased risk of developing breast cancer.

Management Options for Screening and Risk Reduction

Increased Screening

- Annual mammography and breast MRI, alternating every six months, starting at age 30 years
- Clinical breast exam (ideally by a breast surgeon) every 6–12 months, starting at age 25 years
- Monthly breast self-examination starting at age 18 years, with prompt evaluation of any change

Risk-Reducing Surgery

- Bilateral risk-reducing mastectomy with an option of breast reconstruction, for women with a significant family history of breast cancer. Surgery reduces the chance of developing breast cancer by at least 95%.

Age to Test Relatives

- Approximately age 25 years

References

Bowden, A.R., & Tischkowitz, M. (2019). Clinical implications of germline mutations in breast cancer genes: *RECQL*. *Breast Cancer Research and Treatment, 174*(3), 553–560. https://doi.org/10.1007/s10549-018-05096-6

National Comprehensive Cancer Network. (2020). *NCCN Clinical Practice Guidelines in Oncology (NCCN Guidelines®): Genetic/familial high-risk assessment: Breast, ovarian, and pancreatic* [v.2.2021]. https://www.nccn.org/professionals/physician_gls/pdf/genetics_bop.pdf

SMAD4

Cancer Risks

- People with pathogenic variants of *SMAD4* are at risk for developing hamartomatous polyps.
- Incidence of colorectal cancer is 17%–22% by age 35 years and approaches 68% by age 60 years. Median age at diagnosis is 42 years.
- The incidence of gastric cancer is 21% in those with gastric polyps.
- Risk of pancreatic and small bowel cancer may be increased.
- Affected individuals have a risk of hereditary hemorrhagic telangiectasia (HHT), which is associated with epistaxis, telangiectasis, arteriovenous malformations (AVMs), and digital clubbing. Most individuals who have a *SMAD4* germline pathogenic variant have one or more clinical features of HHT.

Management Options for Screening and Risk Reduction

Increased Screening

- Monitoring for rectal bleeding, anemia, abdominal pain, constipation, and diarrhea in childhood
- Colonoscopy and upper endoscopy, starting at approximately age 15 years or earlier if symptoms occur. If no polyps are detected, the screening should be repeated in two to three years. Once polyps are detected, annual screening is indicated.
- Consideration of capsule endoscopy to evaluate for small bowel cancer, starting at approximately age 15 years
- For people with a family history of pancreatic cancer, annual pancreatic screening starting at age 40 years or 10 years prior to the youngest age at pancreatic cancer diagnosis in the family, with MRI/MRCP, EUS, fasting blood glucose, and HbA1c. Annual recommended follow-up includes alternating MRI/MRCP and EUS with annual fasting blood glucose and HbA1c.
- Physical examination, including inspection for telangiectasia (particularly on fingers, lips, tongue, oropharynx, cheeks, or conjunctiva) and listening for abdominal bruits
- Annual complete blood count starting in infancy, with particular attention to anemia or polycythemia. Polycythemia raises suspicion for pulmonary AVMs.
- Contrast echocardiography for detection of pulmonary shunting and AVMs and measurement of the pulmonary artery systolic pressure as a screen for pulmonary artery hypertension.
- MRI of the head with and without gadolinium to detect cerebral AVMs, performed as early as possible, preferably in the first year of life. Adults, including

those screened with MRI in infancy, should have a screening MRI of the head to detect unsuspected vascular lesions and occult cerebral abscesses.
- Consideration of ultrasound or CT examination for evidence of hepatic AVMs, for symptoms such as high-output failure associated with hepatic vascular abnormalities or otherwise unexplained elevations in liver function tests

Risk-Reducing Surgery
- Consideration of colectomy, for an increase in polyps between screening examinations or if malignancy is diagnosed

Other Preventive Measures
- Because of the risks associated with HHT, patients should be instructed to avoid vigorous nose blowing; lifting heavy objects; straining during bowel movements; using electric or chemical cautery for nosebleeds; taking anticoagulant and anti-inflammatory agents, including aspirin, in individuals with significant nose or gastrointestinal bleeding; scuba diving, unless contrast echocardiography within the previous five years was negative for evidence of a right to left shunt; or undergoing liver biopsy.

Age to Test Relatives
- Approximately age one to five years

References

Goggins, M., Overbeek, K.A., Brand, R., Syngal, S., Del Chiaro, M., Bartsch, D.K., ... Bruno, M. (2020). Management of patients with increased risk for familial pancreatic cancer: Updated recommendations from the International Cancer of the Pancreas Screening (CAPS) Consortium. *Gut, 69*(1), 7–17. https://doi.org/10.1136/gutjnl-2019-319352

Larsen Haidle, J., & Howe, J.R. (2017). Juvenile polyposis syndrome. In M.P. Adam, H.H. Ardinger, R.A. Pagon, & S.E. Wallace (Eds.), *GeneReviews®*. University of Washington. https://www.ncbi.nlm.nih.gov/books/NBK1469

McDonald, J., & Pyeritz, R.E. (2017). Hereditary hemorrhagic telangiectasia. In M.P. Adam, H.H. Ardinger, R.A. Pagon, & S.E. Wallace (Eds.), *GeneReviews®*. University of Washington. https://www.ncbi.nlm.nih.gov/books/NBK1351

National Comprehensive Cancer Network. (2020). *NCCN Clinical Practice Guidelines in Oncology (NCCN Guidelines®): Genetic/familial high-risk assessment: Colorectal* [v.1.2020]. https://www.nccn.org/professionals/physician_gls/pdf/genetics_colon.pdf

STK11 (PEUTZ-JEGHERS SYNDROME)

Cancer Risks

- Women with an *STK11* pathogenic variant have the following risks of breast cancer:
  - 8% risk by age 40 years
  - 13% risk age 50 years

  - 31% risk by age 60 years
  - 45% risk by age 70 years
- Lifetime risk of colon cancer is 39%.
- Lifetime risk of stomach cancer is 29%.
- Lifetime risk of small bowel cancer is 13%.
- Lifetime risk of pancreatic cancer is 11%–36%.
- Lifetime risk of developing ovarian cancer is 18%–21%; risk of developing cervical cancer is 10%; and risk of developing endometrial cancer is 9%.
- Risk of testicular cancer is 9%.
- Risk of lung cancer is 7%–17%.

Management Options for Screening and Risk Reduction

Increased Screening

- Annual breast MRI (or mammography if MRI is unavailable) starting at age 25–29 years. At age 30 years and beyond, annual mammography and breast MRI are recommended, alternating every six months.
- Clinical breast exam (ideally by a breast surgeon) every 6–12 months, starting at age 25 years
- Monthly breast self-examination starting at age 18 years, with prompt evaluation of any change
- Upper endoscopy and small bowel examination (magnetic resonance enterography or wireless capsule endoscopy), every one to three years, starting at age eight years or when symptoms occur
- Colonoscopy every one to three years, beginning at age eight years
- In women, gynecologic examination with Pap smear, starting by age 18 years, as well as transvaginal ultrasound and CA-125 testing
- In males, testicular examination and testicular ultrasound, if clinically indicated, starting in childhood
- In men and women, annual pancreatic screening, starting at age 30–35 years or 10 years prior to the youngest age at pancreatic cancer diagnosis in the family, with MRI/MRCP, EUS, fasting blood glucose, and HbA1c. Annual recommended follow-up includes alternating MRI/MRCP and EUS with annual fasting blood glucose and HbA1c.

Risk-Reducing Surgery

- Bilateral risk-reducing mastectomy with an option of breast reconstruction in women with a significant family history of breast cancer. Surgery reduces the chance of developing breast cancer by at least 95%.
- Surgery to remove the ovaries and fallopian tubes at age 40–45 years, when childbearing is complete, in women with a significant family history of gynecologic cancer. Surgery reduces the risk of ovarian cancer by approximately

80%–90%. If surgery occurs before natural menopause, it can reduce the risk of breast cancer by up to 50%.

Age to Test Relatives

- Approximately age three to five years

References

Goggins, M., Overbeek, K.A., Brand, R., Syngal, S., Del Chiaro, M., Bartsch, D.K., ... Bruno, M. (2020). Management of patients with increased risk for familial pancreatic cancer: Updated recommendations from the International Cancer of the Pancreas Screening (CAPS) Consortium. *Gut, 69*(1), 7–17. https://doi.org/10.1136/gutjnl-2019-319352

McGarrity, T.J., Amos, C.I., & Baker, M.J. (2016). Peutz-Jeghers syndrome. In M.P. Adam, H.H. Ardinger, R.A. Pagon, & S.E. Wallace (Eds.), *GeneReviews®*. University of Washington. https://www.ncbi.nlm.nih.gov/books/NBK1266

National Comprehensive Cancer Network. (2020a). *NCCN Clinical Practice Guidelines in Oncology (NCCN Guidelines®): Genetic/familial high-risk assessment: Breast, ovarian, and pancreatic* [v.2.2021]. https://www.nccn.org/professionals/physician_gls/pdf/genetics_bop.pdf

National Comprehensive Cancer Network. (2020b). *NCCN Clinical Practice Guidelines in Oncology (NCCN Guidelines®): Genetic/familial high-risk assessment: Colorectal* [v.1.2020]. https://www.nccn.org/professionals/physician_gls/pdf/genetics_colon.pdf

TP53 (LI-FRAUMENI SYNDROME)

Cancer Risks

- The overall lifetime risk of cancer in individuals with Li-Fraumeni syndrome is 70% or greater for men and 90% or greater for women.
- Adrenocortical carcinomas develop in 6%–13% of affected individuals, with most diagnoses occurring before age five years. It also occurs in adults, typically before age 40 years.
- Women have a 70% lifetime risk of developing breast cancer (12% in the general population).
- The cumulative incidence of brain and neurologic cancer by age 70 years is 6% for women and 19% for men.
- The cumulative incidence of osteosarcomas by age 70 years is 5% for women and 11% for men.
- The cumulative incidence of soft tissue sarcoma is 15% for women and 22% for men, with many occurring before age five years.
- Risk of leukemia is increased.
- Risk of gastrointestinal cancers is increased.
- Although the exact risks are unclear, risk is increased for cancers of the head and neck, kidney, larynx, lung, ovary, pancreas, prostate, testis, and thyroid, as well as melanoma.

Management Options for Screening and Risk Reduction

Increased Screening

- Annual breast MRI (or mammography if MRI is unavailable), starting at age 25–29 years. At age 30 years and beyond, both annual mammography and breast MRI are recommended, alternating every six months.
- Clinical breast exam (ideally by a breast surgeon) every 6–12 months, starting at age 18 years
- Monthly breast self-examination starting at age 18 years, with prompt evaluation of any change
- Comprehensive physical examination and ultrasound of abdomen and pelvis every three to four months from birth to age 18 years
- Annual neurologic exam and whole-body MRI, including brain MRI, from the time of diagnosis
- Upper endoscopy and colonoscopy every two to five years, starting at age 25 years
- For men and women, full body skin examination for melanoma screening starting at age 18 years, with frequency (at least annually) depending on personal and family history of melanoma and atypical moles
- Monthly self-examination of the skin
- For men and women, annual pancreatic screening, starting at age 40 years or 10 years prior to the youngest age at pancreatic cancer diagnosis in the family, with MRI/MRCP, EUS, fasting blood glucose, and HbA1c. Annual recommended follow-up includes alternating MRI/MRCP and EUS with annual fasting blood glucose and HbA1c.

Risk-Reducing Surgery

- Bilateral risk-reducing mastectomy with an option of breast reconstruction. Surgery reduces the chance of developing breast cancer by at least 95%. Surgery also avoids repeated exposure to ionizing radiation with mammography.

Other Preventive Measures

- Affected individuals should minimize exposure to diagnostic and therapeutic radiation.
- Individuals should avoid known carcinogens, including tobacco, occupational exposures, and excessive alcohol use.
- Individuals should avoid artificial tanning.
- When in the sun, individuals should avoid sunburns by using broad-spectrum (UVA/UVB) sunscreen of SPF 30 or higher, seeking shade, covering up with clothing (including hats), and wearing UV-blocking sunglasses.

Age to Test Relatives

- At birth

References

Goggins, M., Overbeek, K.A., Brand, R., Syngal, S., Del Chiaro, M., Bartsch, D.K., ... Bruno, M. (2020). Management of patients with increased risk for familial pancreatic cancer: Updated recommendations from the International Cancer of the Pancreas Screening (CAPS) Consortium. *Gut, 69*(1), 7–17. https://doi.org/10.1136/gutjnl-2019-319352

Kratz, C.P., Achatz, M.I., Brugières, L., Frebourg, T., Garber, J.E., Greer, M.-L.C., ... Malkin, D. (2017). Cancer screening recommendations for individuals with Li-Fraumeni syndrome. *Clinical Cancer Research, 23*(11), e38–e45. https://doi.org/10.1158/1078-0432.CCR-17-0408

National Comprehensive Cancer Network. (2020). *NCCN Clinical Practice Guidelines in Oncology (NCCN Guidelines®): Genetic/familial high-risk assessment: Breast, ovarian, and pancreatic* [v.2.2021]. https://www.nccn.org/professionals/physician_gls/pdf/genetics_bop.pdf

Schneider, K., Zelley, K., Nichols, K.E., & Garber, J. (2019). Li-Fraumeni syndrome. In M.P. Adam, H.H. Ardinger, R.A. Pagon, & S.E. Wallace (Eds.), *GeneReviews®*. University of Washington. https://www.ncbi.nlm.nih.gov/books/NBK1311

VHL (VON HIPPEL-LINDAU SYNDROME)

Cancer Risks

- Individuals with Von Hippel-Lindau syndrome are at increased risk for developing hemangiomas; 80% of hemangiomas develop in the brain and 20% in the spinal cord. Retinal angiomas may develop in childhood.
- Renal cysts are common. Clear cell renal cell carcinoma, developing either within a cyst or in the surrounding parenchyma, occurs in approximately 70% of affected individuals by age 60 years and is a leading cause of death in Von Hippel-Lindau syndrome.
- Risk of benign and malignant pheochromocytoma is increased.
- Risk of benign and malignant paragangliomas is increased.
- Risk of pancreatic cysts is increased. An estimated 5%–17% of individuals with Von Hippel-Lindau syndrome develop neuroendocrine tumors of the pancreas.
- Endolymphatic sac tumors, which result in hearing loss, are seen in approximately 10%–16% of affected individuals.

Management Options for Screening and Risk Reduction

Increased Screening

- Starting at age one year:
  - Annual evaluation for neurologic symptoms, vision problems, or hearing disturbance

- Annual examination for signs of nystagmus, strabismus, or white pupils
- Annual blood pressure monitoring
- Starting at age five years:
  - Annual plasma analysis or 24-hour urine collection for fractionated metanephrines
  - Audiology assessment every two to three years
  - Thin-slice MRI with contrast of the internal auditory canal in those with repeat ear infections
- Starting at age 16 years:
  - Annual abdominal ultrasound
  - MRI of the abdomen, focusing on kidneys, pancreas, and adrenal glands
  - MRI of the brain and total spine every two years

Risk-Reducing Surgery

- No recommendations

Other Preventive Measures

- Individuals should avoid tobacco products because they are considered a risk factor for kidney cancer.
- Chemicals and industrial toxins known to affect Von Hippel-Lindau syndrome–involved organs should be avoided.
- Contact sports should be avoided if adrenal or pancreatic lesions are present.
- Individuals should be educated about the following symptoms, which should be reported and evaluated promptly:
  - High or variable blood pressure, especially spiking blood pressure
  - Increase in frequency or intensity of headaches
  - Increased sweating or what feels like a panic attack, fear, or anxiety
  - Irregular or rapid heartbeat
  - Loss of balance or coordination
  - Loss of bowel or bladder function
  - Loss of hearing
  - Pain (including abdominal pain) of unknown cause

Age to Test Relatives

- At birth

References

Haas, N.B., & Nathanson, K.L. (2014). Hereditary kidney cancer syndromes. *Advances in Chronic Kidney Disease, 21*(1), 81–90. https://doi.org/10.1053/j.ackd.2013.10.001

National Cancer Institute. (2020). Genetics of kidney cancer (renal cell cancer) (PDQ®) [Health professional version]. https://www.cancer.gov/types/kidney/hp/kidney-genetics-pdq

van Leeuwaarde, R.S., Ahmad, S., Links, T.P., & Giles, R.H. (2018). Von Hippel-Lindau syndrome. In M.P. Adam, H.H. Ardinger, R.A. Pagon, & S.E. Wallace (Eds.), *GeneReviews®*. University of Washington. https://www.ncbi.nlm.nih.gov/books/NBK1463

XRCC2

Cancer Risks

- Risk of breast cancer is increased with an *XRCC2* pathogenic variant, but the exact magnitude is unknown.

Management Options for Screening and Risk Reduction

Increased Screening

- Annual mammography starting at approximately age 30 years, with consideration of alternating with breast MRI every six months
- Clinical breast exam (ideally by a breast surgeon) every 6–12 months, starting at age 25 years
- Monthly breast self-examination starting at age 18 years, with prompt evaluation of any change

Risk-Reducing Surgery

- Bilateral risk-reducing mastectomy with an option of breast reconstruction is a consideration for those with a significant family history of breast cancer.

Age to Test Relatives

- Approximately age 25 years

Reference

National Comprehensive Cancer Network. (2020). *NCCN Clinical Practice Guidelines in Oncology (NCCN Guidelines®): Genetic/familial high-risk assessment: Breast, ovarian, and pancreatic* [v.2.2021]. https://www.nccn.org/professionals/physician_gls/pdf/genetics_bop.pdf

Glossary of Terms

allele—One of two or more versions of a gene. An individual inherits two alleles for each gene, one from each parent. If the two alleles are the same, the individual is homozygous for that gene. If the alleles are different, the individual is heterozygous. Although the term *allele* was originally used to describe variation among genes, it now also refers to variation among noncoding DNA sequences.

cascade genetic testing—Process of extending genetic testing to individuals at risk for inheriting a pathogenic variant that was previously identified in a biologic relative. This process is repeated as more pathogenic variant carriers are identified within the family. It is sometimes referred to as *cascade screening* or *cascade testing*, but *cascade genetic testing* is preferred.

chromosome—An organized package of DNA found in the nucleus of the cell. Different organisms have different numbers of chromosomes. Humans have 23 pairs of chromosomes—22 pairs of numbered chromosomes, called autosomes, and one pair of sex chromosomes, X and Y. Each parent contributes one chromosome to each pair in offspring.

consanguinity—Kinship characterized by the sharing of common ancestors.

deoxyribonucleic acid (DNA)—Basic unit of heredity that is the carrier of genetic information. The billions of nucleotides are organized linearly along the double helix in functional units known as *genes*.

DNA bases—The four types of nitrogen bases are adenine (A), thymine (T), guanine (G), and cytosine (C). The order of these bases determines DNA's instructions, or genetic code.

founder effect—The reduced genetic diversity in an ethic group that results when a population is descended from a small number of ancestors. The resulting population may be very different from the original population, both in terms of its genotypes and phenotypes.

gene—The basic unit of heredity. A gene occupies a specific location on a chromosome. Each gene consists of nucleotides arranged in a linear manner. Most genes code for a specific protein or segment of protein leading to a particular characteristic or function.

genetics—The study of genes and heredity.

genomics—The study of the entire genome, which includes all the genes that can be found in an organism.

genotype—An individual's collection of genes. The term can also refer to the two alleles inherited for a particular gene. The genotype is expressed when the information encoded in the genes' DNA is used to make protein and RNA molecules. The expression of the genotype contributes to the individual's observable traits, known as the *phenotype.*

germline—The sex cells (eggs and sperm) used by sexually reproducing organisms to pass on genes from generation to generation. Egg and sperm cells are known as *germ cells*, whereas the other cells of the body, known as *somatic cells.*

Gleason score—Description of how abnormal the cancer cells in a prostate biopsy sample appear and how quickly they are likely to grow and spread. Most prostate cancers contain cells that are different grades. The Gleason score is calculated by adding together the two grades of cancer cells that make up the largest areas of the biopsied tissue sample. The Gleason score usually ranges from 6 to 10. A lower Gleason score indicates that more cancer cells appear similar to healthy cells and are likely to grow and spread slowly. The Gleason score is used to help plan treatment and determine prognosis.

hereditary cancer syndrome—A type of inherited disorder in which a person has a greater risk of certain types of cancer than the general population. Hereditary cancer syndromes are caused by pathogenic variants (sometimes referred to as *mutations*) in certain genes passed from parents to children.

heredity—The passing of genetic information and traits, such as hair or eye color or an increased probability of developing a certain disease, from parents to offspring.

heterozygous—Having inherited different alleles of a particular gene from each parent. A heterozygous genotype stands in contrast to a homozygous genotype, in which an individual inherits identical forms of a particular gene from each parent.

homozygous—Genetic condition in which an individual inherits the same alleles for a particular gene from both parents.

likely pathogenic variant—A genetic variant very likely to contribute to the development of disease, but scientific evidence is currently insufficient to prove this conclusively.

microsatellite instability (MSI)—Microsatellite sequences are repetitive DNA sequences usually several base pairs in length. They are used as genetic markers to follow the inheritance of genes in families. A characteristic of cells that contain an abnormality in DNA mismatch repair is referred to as *microsatellite instability.* Microsatellite testing that shows alterations or errors in 30% or more of microsatellites is termed as *microsatellite instability-high.* Microsatellite instability-high cancer cells may have a defect in their ability to correct mistakes that occur when DNA is copied in the cell. Microsatellite instability is found most often in colorectal, gastric, and endometrial cancers, but it may also be found in many other cancers.

mosaicism—The presence of two or more populations of cells with different genotypes in one individual who has developed from a fertilized egg.

mutation—A variant in the structure of the gene that is pathogenic or likely pathogenic. This is an older term synonymous with *pathogenic variant*, which is the preferred term. See also *pathogenic variant* or *likely pathogenic variant.*

next-generation sequencing (NGS)—High-throughput method used to determine a portion of the nucleotide sequence of an individual's genome. This technique utilizes DNA sequencing technologies that are capable of processing multiple DNA sequences in parallel. It is also known as *massively parallel sequencing.*

nomenclature—A system of names, terms, or rules for forming these terms in a particular field of arts or sciences. In genetics, gene nomenclature is the scientific naming of genes, the units of heredity in living organisms.

noninformative negative result—A genetic testing result occurring when the first person tested in a family does not have a pathogenic variant.

panel testing—A form of genetic testing that looks for changes in many genes in one test. Panel genetic tests can also be grouped into genes that are all associated with higher risk of developing certain kinds of cancer, such as breast or colorectal cancer.

pathogenic variant—Change in the genetic material that directly contributes to the development of disease. Additional evidence is not expected to alter the classification of this variant. Historically, a pathogenic variant is also known as a *mutation.* Not all pathogenic variants are fully penetrant.

pedigree—An illustration of genetic family history that diagrams the inheritance of a trait or disease though several generations. A pedigree shows the relationships between family members and indicates which individuals express or silently carry the trait in question.

penetrance—The likelihood that a clinical condition will occur when a particular genotype is present. For adult-onset diseases, penetrance is usually described by the individual carrier's age, sex, and organ site.

phenotype—The observable characteristics in an individual resulting from the expression of genes; the clinical presentation of an individual with a particular genotype.

polygenic risk score—Assessment of the risk of a specific condition based on the collective influence of many genetic variants. These can include variants associated with genes of known function and variants not known to be associated with genes relevant to the condition.

polymorphism—One of multiple variants of a particular DNA sequence. The most common type of polymorphism involves variation at a single base pair known as a *single nucleotide polymorphism* (SNP; pronounced "snip"). Polymorphisms can also be much larger in size and involve long stretches of DNA.

positive result—Result occurring when a genetic test identifies a pathogenic or likely pathogenic variant that increases the risk for developing cancer.

precision medicine—A form of medicine that uses information about a person's own genes or proteins to prevent, diagnose, or treat disease. In oncology, precision medicine uses specific information about a person's tumor to help make a diagnosis, plan treatment, determine how treatment is working, or make a prognosis. It is also known as *personalized medicine.*

proband—An individual being studied or reported on in a genetic study. A proband is usually the first affected individual in a family who brings a genetic disorder to the attention of healthcare providers and is the starting point for the genetic study of a family.

Sanger DNA sequencing—A low-throughput method of DNA sequencing used to determine a portion of the nucleotide sequence of an individual's genome. This technique uses polymerase chain reaction (PCR) amplification of genetic regions of interest followed by sequencing of PCR products. The Sanger method only sequences a single DNA fragment at a time.

sequencing—Process that determines the order of the four chemical building blocks (adenine, thymine, guanine, and cytosine) that make up the DNA molecule.

single nucleotide polymorphism (SNP)—A DNA sequence variation that occurs when a single nucleotide (adenine, thymine, cytosine, or guanine) in the genome sequence is altered; usually present in at least 1% of the population.

somatic—Any cell of the body except sperm and egg cells. Somatic cells are diploid, meaning that they contain two sets of chromosomes, one inherited from each parent. Pathogenic variants in somatic cells can affect the individual, but they are not passed on to offspring.

triple-negative breast cancer—Breast cancer that tests negative for estrogen receptors, progesterone receptors, and excess HER2 protein. These results indicate that the growth of the malignancy is not stimulated by the hormones estrogen and progesterone or by the HER2 protein.

true negative result—For families in which members have a known pathogenic variant, a test result that shows an individual has not inherited the pathogenic variant.

variable expressivity—Degree or variation to which a genotype is expressed.

variant—An alteration in the most common DNA nucleotide sequence. The term *variant* can be used to describe an alteration that may be benign, pathogenic, or of unknown significance. Variants may be germline or somatic. The term is increasingly being used in place of *mutation.*

variant of unknown significance—Genetic test result of a detected change in the genetic material, but it is not clear if the change is harmless or harmful.

zygote—Fertilized ovum that forms the first cell in a human.

For more genetic terms, please refer to the ONS Genomics Taxonomy (www.ons.org/genomics-taxonomy).

BIBLIOGRAPHY

National Cancer Institute. (n.d.). *NCI dictionary of cancer terms.* https://www.cancer.gov/publications/dictionaries/cancer-terms

National Cancer Institute. (n.d.). *NCI dictionary of genetic terms.* https://www.cancer.gov/publications/dictionaries/genetics-dictionary

National Cancer Institute. (2020, July 24). *Cancer genetics overview (PDQ®)* [Health professional version]. https://www.cancer.gov/about-cancer/causes-prevention/genetics/overview-pdq

National Human Genome Research Institute. (n.d.). *Talking glossary of genetics terms.* https://www.genome.gov/genetics-glossary

Index

The letter *f* after a page number indicates that relevant content appears in a figure; the letter *t*, in a table.

C

D

E

F

G

H

S

T

U

V

X

Z